K. Morgenroth
M.T. Newhouse

BRONCHITIS

Drawings:
G. Pucher

Pharmazeutische Verlagsgesellschaft

BUTTERWORTH SCIENTIFIC
LONDON · BOSTON · SINGAPORE · SYDNEY · WELLINGTON · DURBAN · TORONTO

Authors:

Prof. Dr. Konrad Morgenroth
Institut für Pathologie der Ruhr-Universität Bochum
Universitätsstraße 150
4630 Bochum 1

Dr. Michael T. Newhouse
M.D.C.M., M. Sc., F.R.C.P. (C), F.A.C.P.
Clinical Professor of Medicine, McMaster University
Head Firestone Regional Chest and Allergy Unit, St. Joseph's Hospital
50 Charlton Avenue East
Hamilton, Ontario L8N 1Y4
Canada

ISBN 3-88581-043-3
English Language Edition Published by Butterworth Scientific Ltd
ISBN 0407 002 790
Translation: H.P. Schleiss
Original version: ISBN 3-88581-039-5
PVG Pharmazeutische Verlagsgesellschaft mbH

Preface

Bronchitis is one of the most common conditions seen in the practice of medicine. Patients with this condition must frequently be followed and treated for many years. In recent years, numerous epidemiological investigations have been undertaken which have attempted to evaluate the role of personal and environmental pollutants in the aetiology and pathogenesis of bronchitis.

During the past 30 years, sophisticated methods of evaluating pulmonary function have provided an increased understanding of the pathophysiology of bronchitis. Furthermore, the fiberoptic bronchoscope has allowed the Clinician to assess the morphology of the bronchial mucosa more readily and relate this to the clinical and physiological state of the patient.

Because of the ease with which fiberoptic bronchoscopy can be performed, serial biopsies of the mucosa make it possible for the Pathologist to provide information about the evolution of the disease while at the same time improvement or deterioration of physiological variables and clinical features can be monitored.

This book attempts to improve our understanding of the clinical, pathophysiological and pathological features of bronchitis by means of photobronchography, light and electron microscopy and the superb drawings of graphic artist Gerhard Pucher. We are particularly grateful to Docent Dr. J. Nakhosteen for his excellent photobronchographs.

We would also like to thank the Editor, Mr. Klaus Jarosch and Pharmazeutische Verlagsgesellschaft for the numerous superb graphics which helped to provide a comprehensive picture of this common condition.

Bochum, Germany, K. Morgenroth

Hamilton, Canada, M. Newhouse

Table of Contents

1. Introduction

The term "bronchitis" encompasses all of the inflammatory changes of the bronchial tree.

Respiratory diseases are amongst the most frequent afflictions of man and bronchitis is one of the most important causes of morbidity and mortality due to respiratory disease. Even in patients dying of innumerable other conditions, bronchitis is often an incidental finding at post mortem.

The chief aetiological factors predisposing to bronchitis include tobacco smoking, infections, allergic reactions, aspiration of refluxed gastric contents and, to a much lesser degree, occupational and environmental air pollution.

A study published in 1975 by the German Research Council detailed the factors predisposing to the development of chronic obstructive and nonobstructive bronchitis including such things as smoking and occupational dust exposure as well as many other contributing causes such as age, constitutional predisposition, climate, allergic sensitization and environmental gases and particulates in highly polluted industrialized areas.

The fact that only a minority of people living in such areas develops chronic bronchitis has led to the conclusion that it must be the combination of genetic predisposition and inhaled pollutants that results in the development of airway disease in nonsmokers.

Acute and chronic bronchitis should be distinguished in terms of aetiology, clinical presentation, pathology, pathophysiology, therapy, course and particularly prognosis resulting from the inflammatory changes of the bronchial tree.

The most important functional sequela of bronchitis is airway obstruction characterized by an increase in airway flow resistance usually associated with pulmonary hyperinflation. There may or may not be associated pulmonary emphysema and the condition may progress, usually over many years, to cardio-pulmonary insufficiency and chronic pulmonary heart disease. Regardless of aetiology, the end stage of the disease is similar.

In general it is very difficult and in the individual case quite impossible to demonstrate a specific relationship between various inhaled pollutants determined from the history and individual components of the pathological picture. Since chronic bronchitis is only one part of the disease complex, it has become clinical practice to speak of chronic obstructive airway disease.

The increased application of bronchoscopy in recent years has contributed to an improved understanding of the morphology of the disease. Evaluation of pathological changes has contributed immeasurably to our understanding of the structure and function of the bronchial mucosa and its changes in inflammatory reactions. An understanding of morphology of bronchitis has also contributed to an improved understanding of the clinical picture and evaluation of response to therapy.

The microscopic changes of acute and chronic bronchitis are reflected in the endoscopic appearance. Typical macroscopic features can be seen in the trachea and bronchi. The demonstration of bronchoscopic and histological features of bronchitis down to electron microscopic dimensions should contribute considerably to an understanding of the clinical picture.

Fig. 1: Schematic representation of transnasal fiberoptic bronchoscopy showing the tip of the bronchoscope positioned just above the vocal cords. The transnasal route allows the bronchoscope to be introduced readily with minimum patient discomfort.

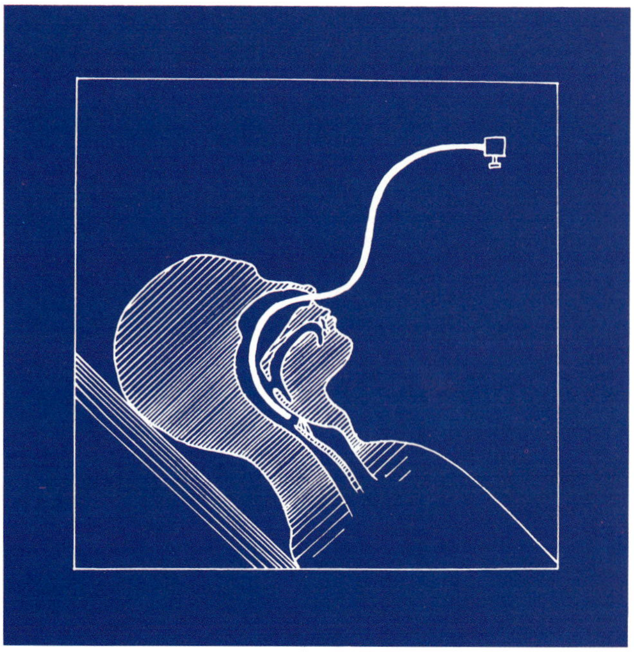

By starting with the normal structure of the bronchial mucosa and evaluating the individual characteristic morphological features of bronchitis, it should be possible to construct a clear picture of the structural changes resulting from chronic airway inflammation. An improved understanding of the morphological features should lead to improved insight into the functional abnormalities.

Bronchoscopy

Bronchoscopy was usually performed in patients over the age of 40, in whom increasing cough, persistent pulmonary infiltrates or an obvious mass lesion on chest roentgenography demanded exclusion of bronchogenic carcinoma.

The photobronchographs were taken by Docent Dr. J. Nakhosteen at the Ruhrlandklinik, Essen, Germany. The fiberoptic bronchoscope-system consisted of an Olympus fiberoptic bronchoscope (B.F. 6C, Olympus O.M. 2 camera) and magnification adapter (SM 4S) manufactured by the Olympus Optical Company, Tokyo. The endoscope has a high degree of resolution similar to the Hopkin's Optics previously used for rigid bronchoscopy. All bronchoscopies were performed using topical anaesthesia. The majority of photographs were obtained by placing the tip of the fiberoptic bronchoscope 3 cm below the vocal cords (Fig. 1). The use of topical anaesthesia made it possible to observe respiratory tract dynamics over prolonged periods. In advanced bronchitis, airway dynamics were frequently seen to be impaired.

In order to demonstrate progression from the normal to acute inflammatory change and from recurrent acute inflammatory changes to chronic bronchitis, photographs of the tracheal mucosa have been used. The progression of the gross abnormalities seen through the bronchoscope consist of:

- Thickening and coarsening of the mucosa as a result of hypertrophy of various mucosal components (mucus glands, basement membrane, etc).
- Mucus hypersecretion.
- Increasing airway collapse resulting from loss of elasticity of the pars membranacea, occasionally tracheomalacia as well as increased compressive forces and the Bernoulli effect.

Histological Material

Most of the histological studies were undertaken on biopsy specimens obtained at bronchoscopy. In addition, post mortem material and material from animal studies was also used.

Electron Microscopy

Great care was taken in the handling of the biopsy material which was immediately placed in 3% gluteraldehyde in phosphate buffer or formalin to achieve optimal preservation of tissue.

Light Microscopy (LM)

Light microscopy was undertaken with the orthoplan Leitz microscope with orthomat attachment.

Scanning Electron Photomicrography (SEM)

Was performed by means of the Leitz AMR 1000 microscope. The pathological material was prepared using the critical point drying technique.

Transmission Electron Photomicrography (TEM)

Photographs were obtained by means of the Zeiss EM 109 microscope. Material was embedded in epon and stained by means of lead citrate and uranyl acetate.

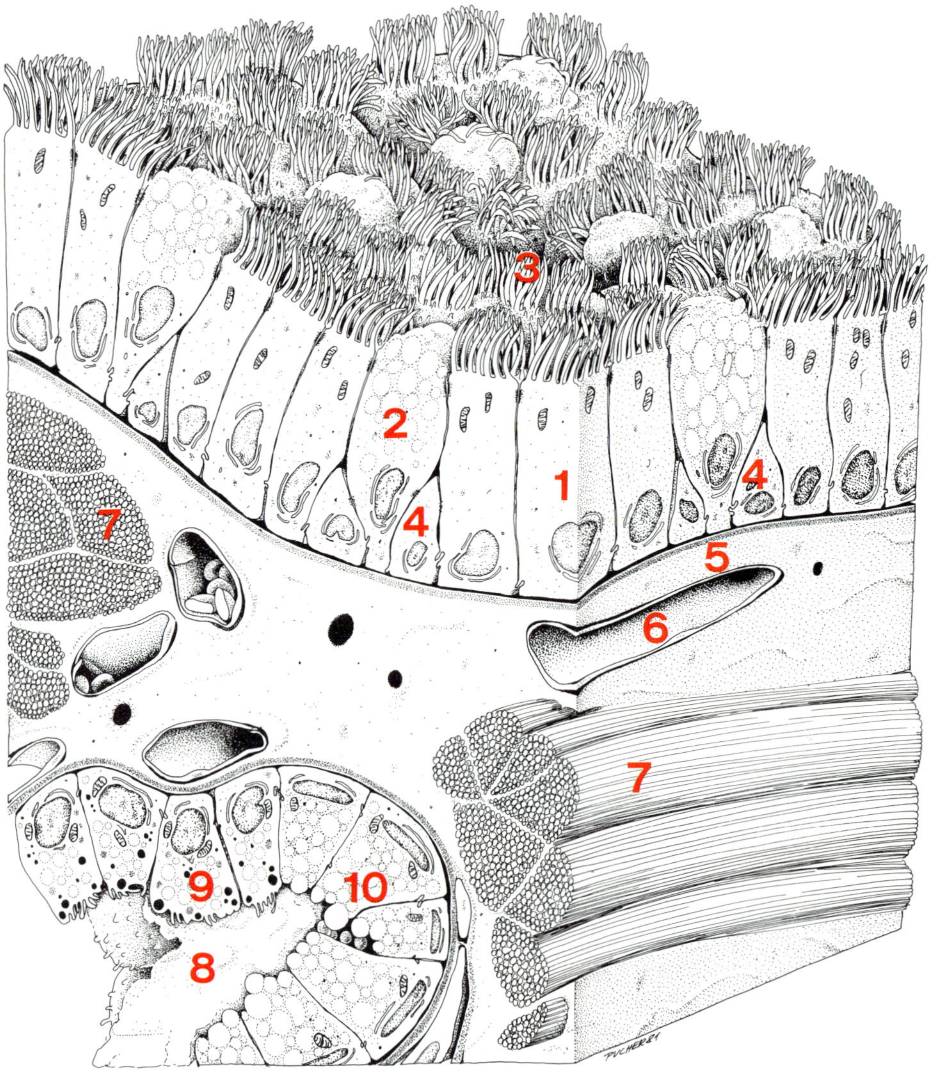

Fig. 2: Three dimensional diagram showing features of the normal bronchial mucosa.

1: ciliated cells
2: goblet cells
3: peribronchial gland duct orifice on the epithelial surface
4: basal cell of the bronchial epithelium
5: basal lamella
6: subepithelial vasculature surrounded by connective tissue
7: smooth muscle of the bronchial wall
8: peribronchial gland
9: serous epithelial cells
10: mucous epithelial cells

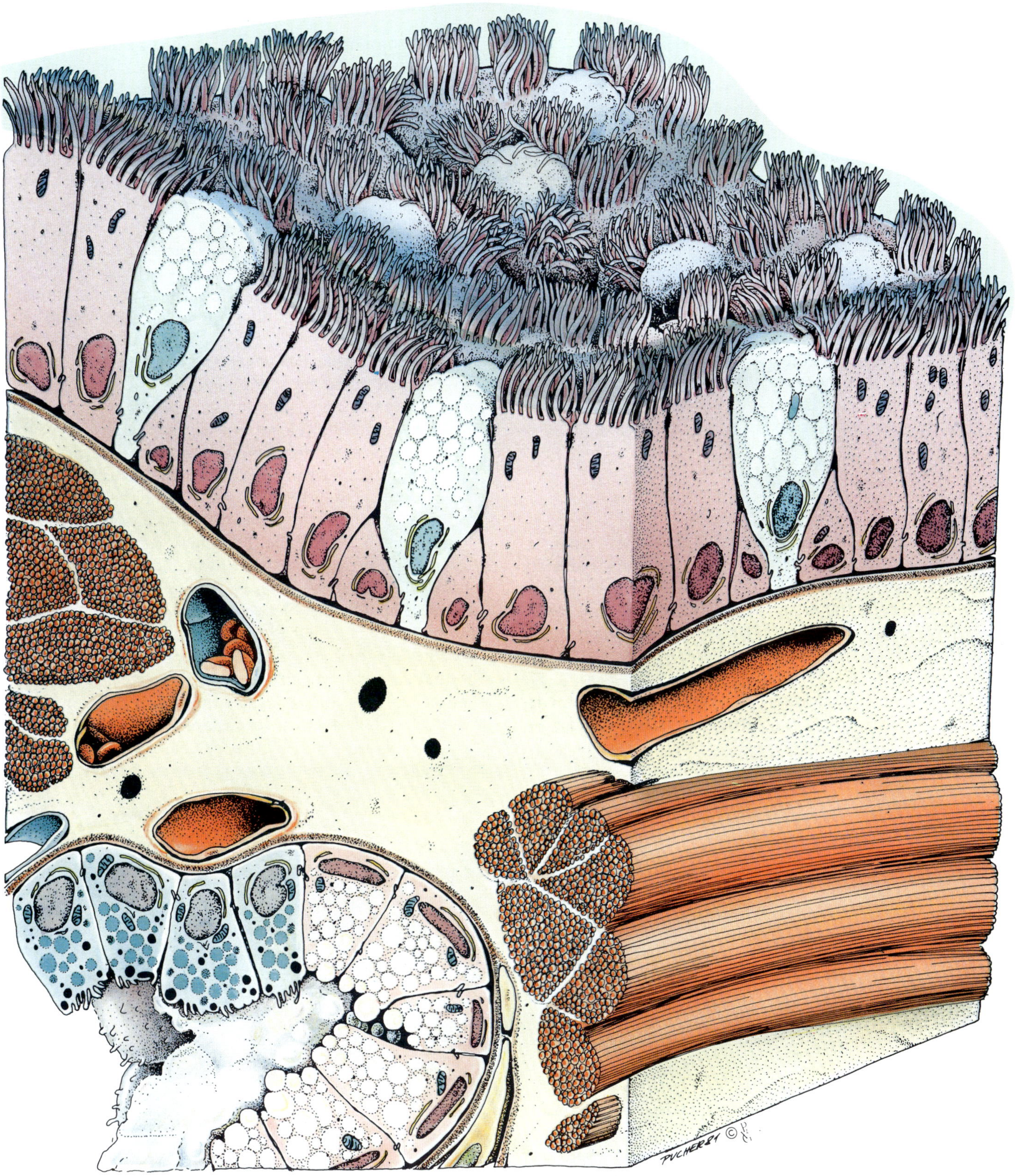

2. Morphology of the Bronchial Tree

The bronchial tree divides dichotomously and only rarely into three branches up to 16-fold. The diameter of the airway decreases from 1.5 to 2.0cm in the trachea to 0.5mm in the terminal bronchioles. Tracheal patency is maintained by 16-20 horseshoe-shaped cartilaginous rings. In the mainstem bronchi, these become cartilaginous plates. Distal of the segmental bronchi, the cartilaginous tissue disappears to be replaced by a fibroblastic fibrous tunica which becomes progressively thinner as it extends towards the prelobular bronchi.

The bronchial wall contains smooth muscle arranged in a lattice-like arrangement. In the trachea, this smooth muscle extends between the free ends of the cartilaginous rings while in the cartilage-containing bronchi, it forms rings of smooth muscle which become thicker in more peripheral airways. Distal to the prelobular bronchi the smooth muscle helps to stabilize the tubular airway system.

The bronchi are supplied with blood via the bronchial arteries which run in the peribronchial tissue to the level of subsegmental bronchi. More distally, they separate from the bronchial wall and travel in the inferior lobular septae to the visceral pleura. Their blood flows into the bronchial veins, pulmonary capillaries and pleural capillaries. Short bronchopulmonary arterial anastomoses result in arteriovenous shunts in some disease states.

The lung is innervated by the vagus and sympathetic systems which run in the peribronchial tissue and synapse in autonomic ganglia which also lie in the peribronchial tissue. Post-ganglionic fibres innervate airway and vascular smooth muscle. The bronchial mucosa provides a continuous fluid covering consisting of a sol-like periciliary fluid layer above which floats a gel-like mucus blanket. This blanket is probably discontinuous in more peripheral airways and continuous in the trachea and major bronchi. By means of mucociliary transport, the continuously secreted mucus is transported from peripheral to more central airways at linear velocities ranging from 0.1 mm/min in the terminal bronchiole to approximately 1 cm/min in the trachea. Finally, secretions are transported into the pharynx to be swallowed. The airway mucosa provides a humidification function to prevent the subjacent tissue from becoming dehydrated while at the same time providing an effective barrier against organic and inorganic substances inhaled with the large volumes of air necessary to accomplish gas exchange. Additional lung defences include lysozyme and other humoral factors in the bronchial mucus and periciliary fluid, the bronchial mucosal epithelium, subepithelial immuno-competent cells and mucus from the glands which lie in the bronchial submucosa. The trachea and bronchi are lined throughout by a pseudostratified, ciliated columnar epithelium interspersed with goblet cells. These goblet cells are present in a ratio of 1:5 in the trachea but in more peripheral airways they become less frequent and are virtually absent in the normal terminal bronchiole. In addition to ciliated cells and goblet cells, the bronchial epithelium also contains basal cells from which the former are derived.

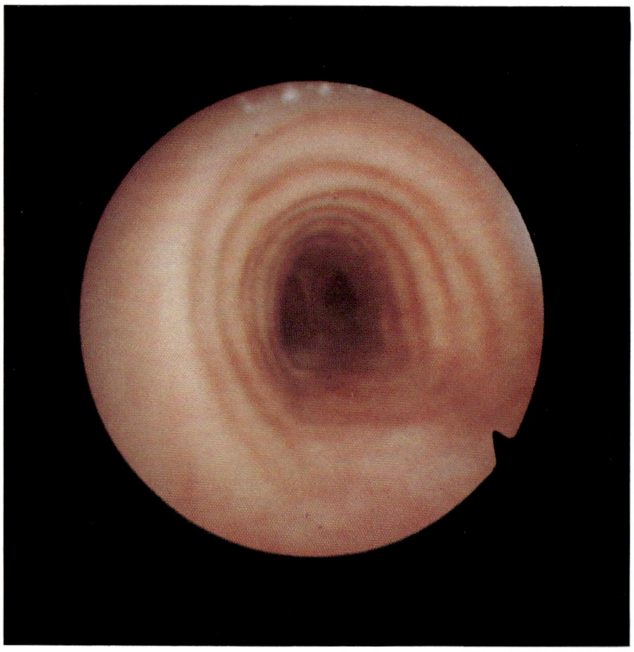

Fig. 3: Photograph of the normal tracheal mucosa seen through the bronchoscope.
The longitudinally arranged fibres of the pars membranacea join the horseshoe-shaped cartilaginous rings on either side. The mucosa shows a smooth surface and is covered by a thin mucous layer.

Fig. 4: Microscopic appearance of the subepithelial connective tissue of the bronchial wall.
The blood and lymphatic vessels and nerve fibres supplying the bronchial mucosa are seen, surrounded by the loose submucosal connective tissue.

Light microscopy (LM)
Semi-thin section
Stain: Basic fuchsin and methylene blue
Magnification: 1,200:1

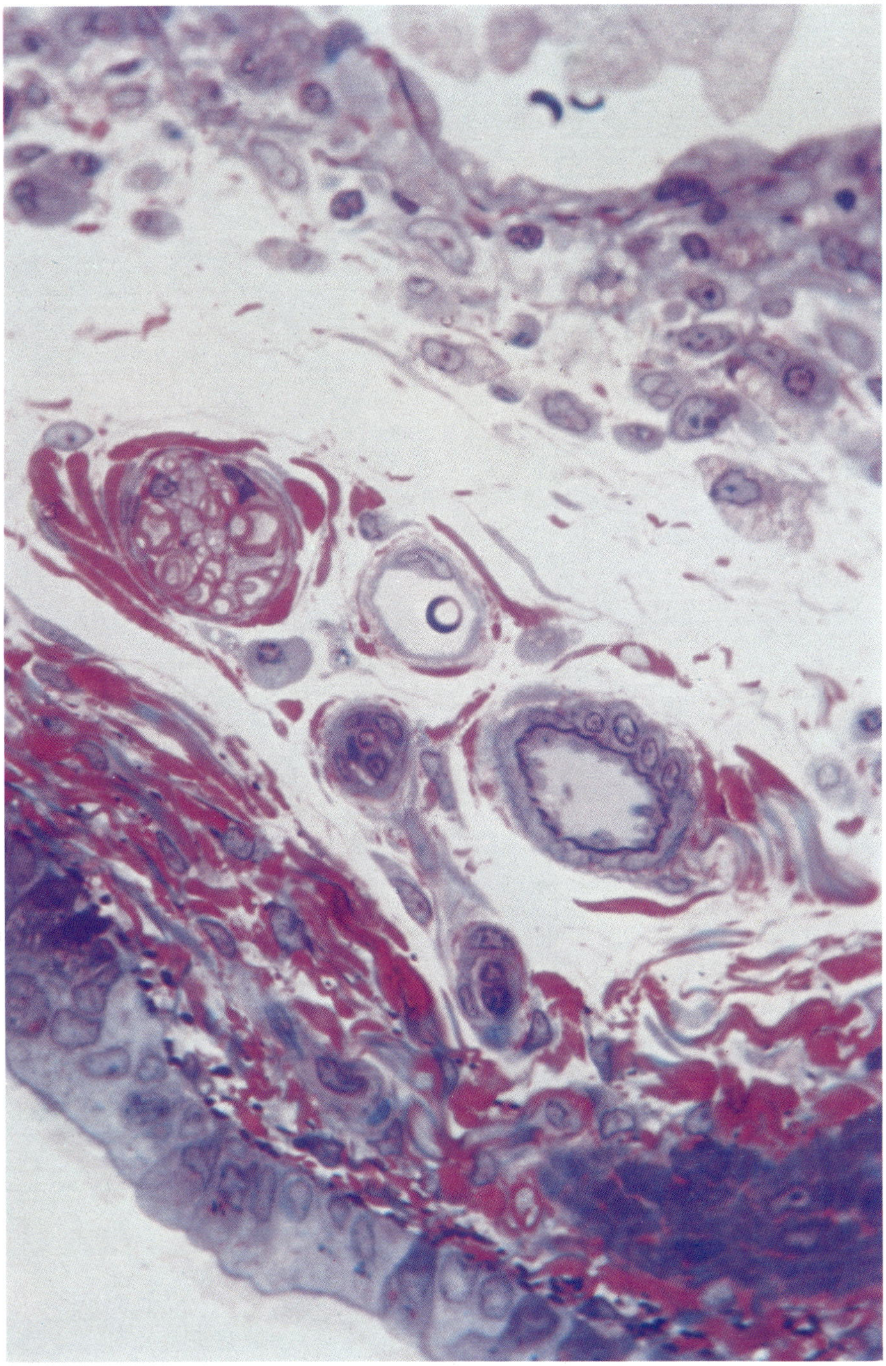

2.1. Basal Cells

The basal cells are located on the basal lamella and do not extend to the epithelial surface. They are most often pyramidal in shape with their base on the basal lamella and their apex directed towards the epithelial surface. The basal cells are connected to one another and adjacent columnar cells by means of interdigitations of their cell membrane and desmosomes. Desmosomes are well defined contact zones of two neighbouring cell membranes with a diameter of approximately 0.5 μm. Each adjacent cell contributes half a desmosome to establish the area of contact. At these sites, the cell membranes are thickened and the adjacent cytoplasm is more dense. Fine tono-filaments run from the areas of increased density into the cytoplasm. The space between the two

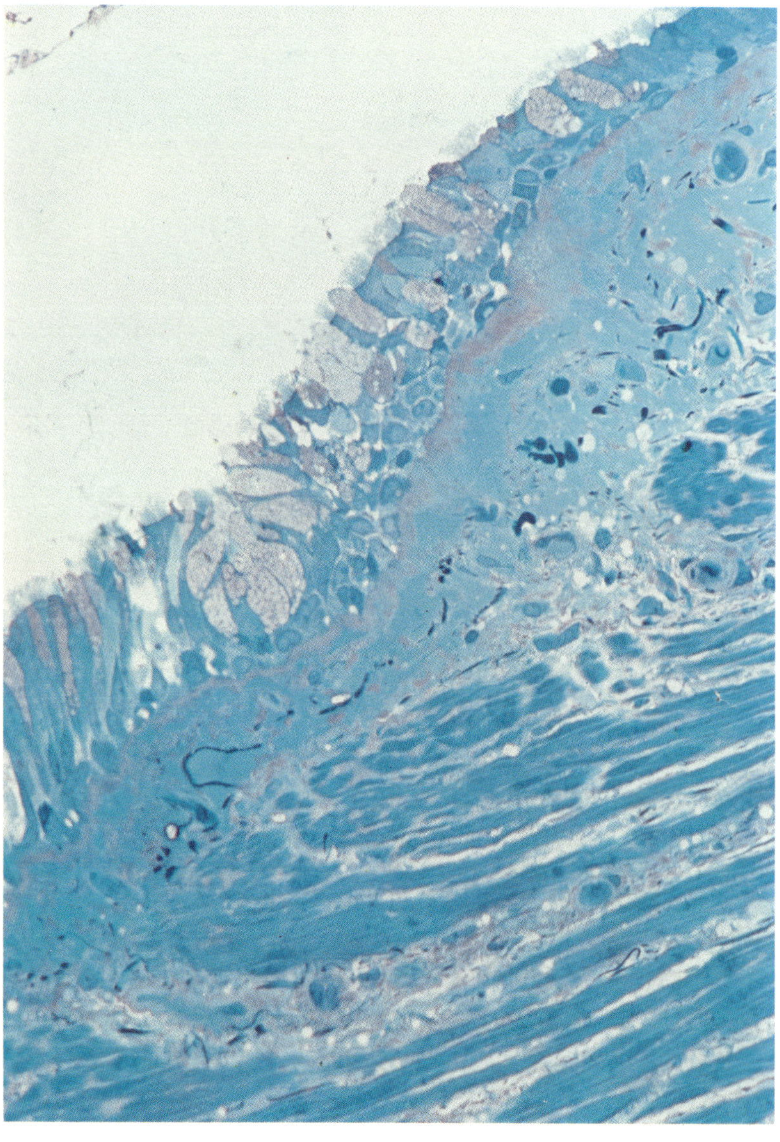

Fig. 5: Histological appearance of the bronchial mucosa.
Pseudostratified ciliated columnar epithelium. The epithelium shows ciliated and goblet cells in a ratio of 5:1. The subepithelial connective tissue contains blood and lymph vessels and small strips of smooth muscle.

Semi-thin section
Stain: Basic fuchsin and methylene blue
Magnification: 520:1

half-desmosomes is probably filled with a cement substance rich in polysaccharides. The desmosomes stick the epithelium together and may also play a role in transmitting information from cell to cell. Furthermore, hemi-desmosomes appear to provide a point of contact between the basal cells and the basal lamella.

The nuclei of the basal cells are round or ellipsoid and fill most of the cell. There are relatively few cytoplasmic organelles. The cytoplasm contains a large number of fine tono-filaments which traverse the cell in different directions and often converge at the desmosomes. The basal cells are the undifferentiated cells of the bronchial epithelium from which ciliated and goblet cells arise.

Fig. 6: Cross section of bronchial epithelium.
The epithelium consists of slender cells attached to the basal lamella by their narrow base. Between these cells, there are pyramidal basal cells. The cilia of the ciliated cells have a tufted appearance. The goblet cells contain clear intracytoplasmic secretory granules.

Transmission electron photomicrograph (TEM)
Magnification 1,700:1

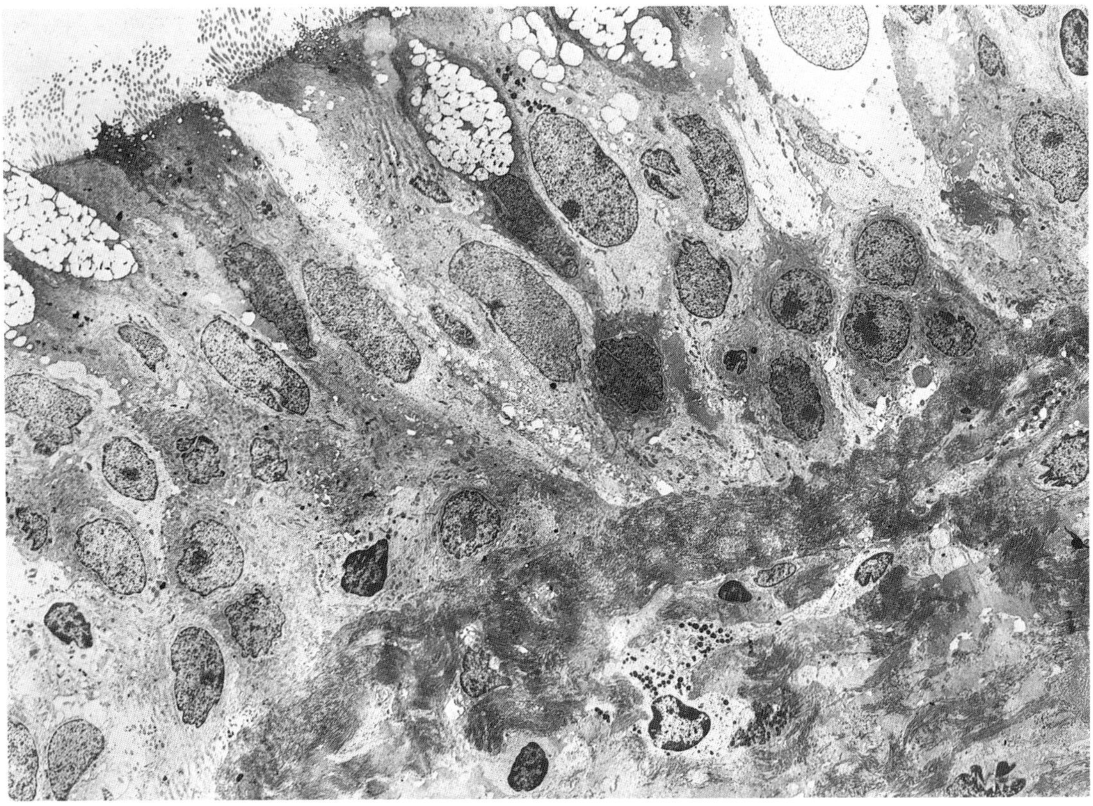

2.2. Ciliated Cells

Of all the mucosal cells in the trachea and bronchi, ciliated cells are most common. They extend from the basal lamella, between the basal cells to the epithelial surface. Their oval nucleus is located at the base of the cell just above the basal cell layer. Their cytoplasm is loosely arranged and of low electron density and contains widely scattered ribosomes some of which are clustered together. The endoplasmic reticulum is not well developed. A perinuclear Golgi apparatus is sometimes seen and mitochondria are numerous. These are located predominantly at the apex of the ciliated cell just below the basal bodies of the cilia. They have an elongated, somewhat branching appearance. Numerous parallel oriented cristae extend from the edge into their matrix. The mitochondria presumably serve to provide the adenosine triphosphate (ATP) required for ciliary motility. In the cytoplasm of the ciliated cells, there are lysosomes whose function is not fully understood. They might be autophagolysosomes which function to break down cytoplasmic debris by means of lysosomal enzymes.

Cilia cover the surface of ciliated cells. These motile portions of the cytoplasm have a uniform length of approximately 5 μm and are 0.2-0.3 μm wide. The ciliary mem-

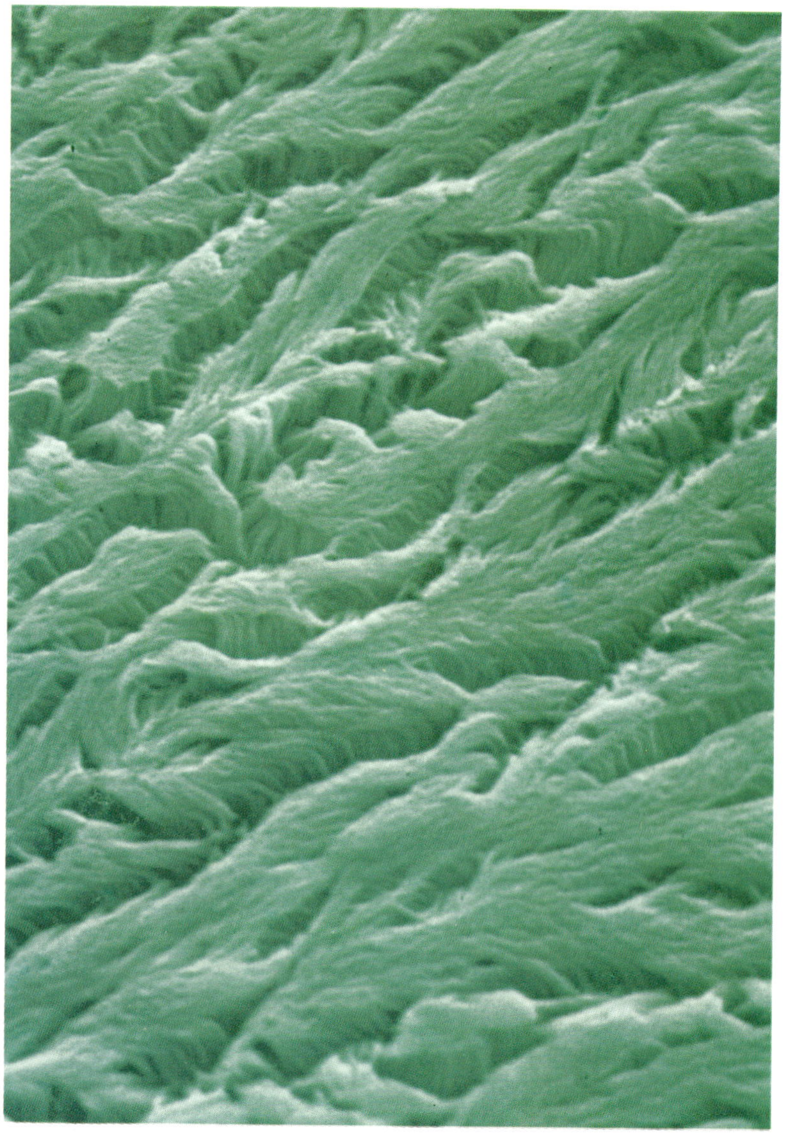

Fig. 7: Surface epithelium of the bronchial mucosa with uniform, densely packed cilia. The cilia beat in metachronal waves.

Scanning electron photomicrograph (SEM)
Magnification: 1,200:1

brane is an extension of the cell membrane. Between the cilia, arising from the surface of the ciliated cells, there are finger-like branching thin cytoplasmic protrusions called microvillae.

Ciliary ultrastructure is remarkably identical throughout the animal kingdom and consists of two central microtubules surrounded by nine peripheral micro-tubular doublets. The paired central tubules are surrounded by a helical sheath. The peripheral doublets consist of a cylindrical subfibre A to which is attached a crescentic subfibre B. The central and peripheral microtubules are connected to one another by means of radial spokes and the peripheral doublets are interconnected via nexin links and dynein arms. The dynein arms are small hook-like projections attached to the subfibre A which appear to become connected to the subfibre B of the adjacent doublet during ciliary motion. The outer dynein arm is somewhat larger than the inner one. Dynein arms are arranged periodically like rungs of a ladder between the base and apex of the subfibre A of the microtubular doublet. While the peripheral microtubules appear to originate in the basal body of the ciliated cell, the central microtubules originate in the lower third of the cilium

Fig. 8: Surface of the bronchial mucosa.
Goblet cells are seen interspersed between ciliated cells in an early stage of the secretory cycle. Microvilli are distributed regularly over the surface of the goblet cells. The goblet cells are surrounded by cilia.

SEM
Magnification: 2,500:1

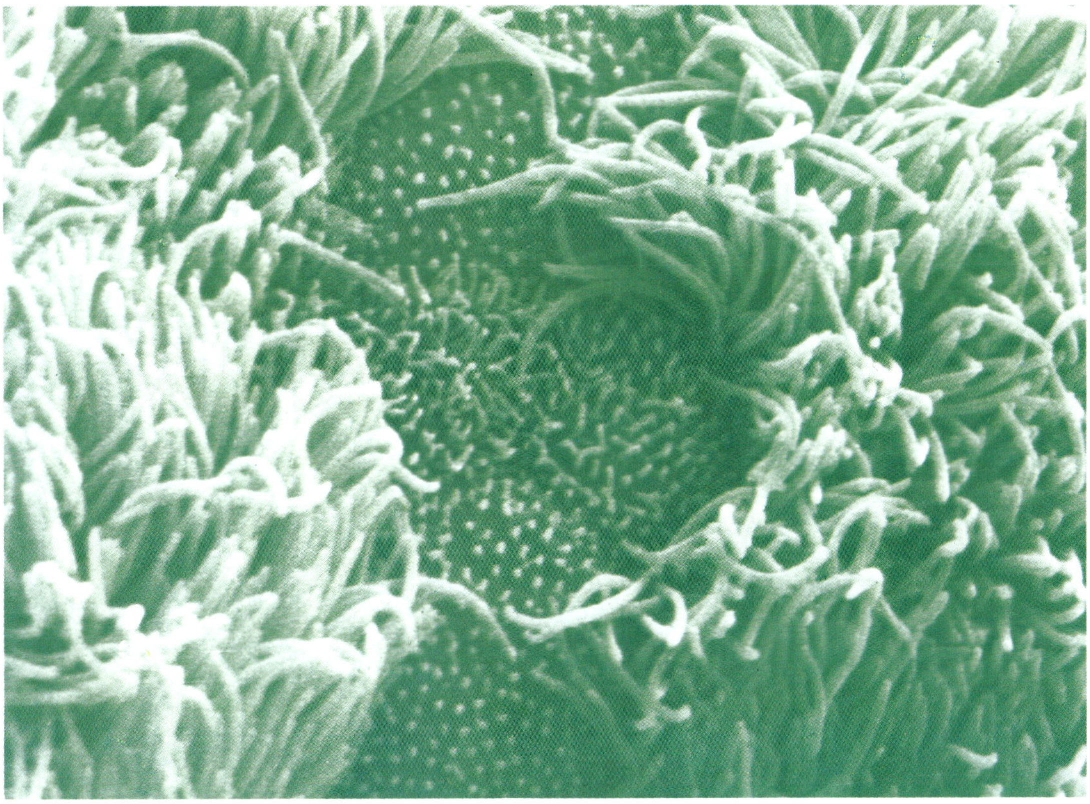

Fig. 9: Cross section of cilia.
The ultrastructure of the axoneme is shown sectioned at different levels. There is a characteristic 9 + 2 arrangement of the microtubules. The centre of the axoneme contains paired microtubules which travel longitudinally from the lower third of the cilium to the tip. Radial spokes join the central microtubules to the nine peripheral doublets. Small hook-like dynein arms are attached to one of the tubules of the peripheral doublets. The orientation of the central tubules is quite uniform from lower left to upper right in the photograph indicating the direction of ciliary beating. Between the ciliated cells are vesicular structures outlined by a fine phospholipid lamella.

TEM
Magnification: 48,000:1

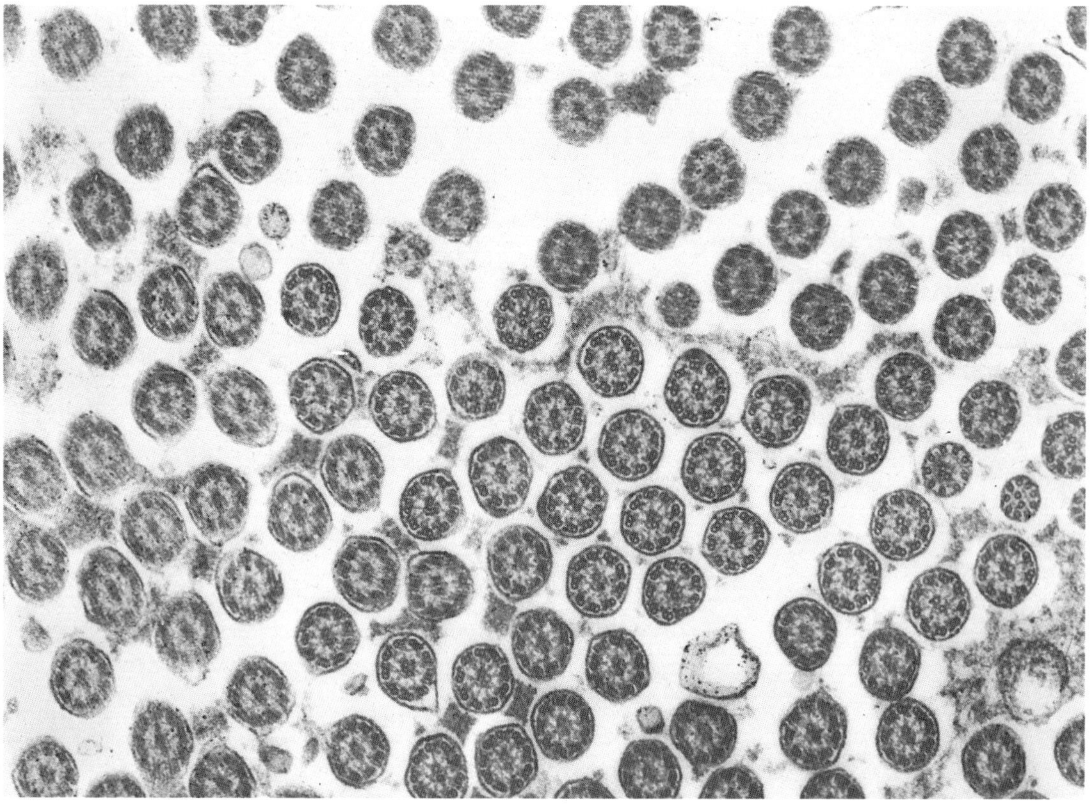

Fig. 10: Cilia in longitudinal section.
Cilia taper towards a dome-shaped tip. Between the tips of the cilia are fine floccular secretions. At the extreme tip of the cilium are filamentous projections (inset).

TEM
Magnification: 30,000:1
Magnification (inset): 90,000:1

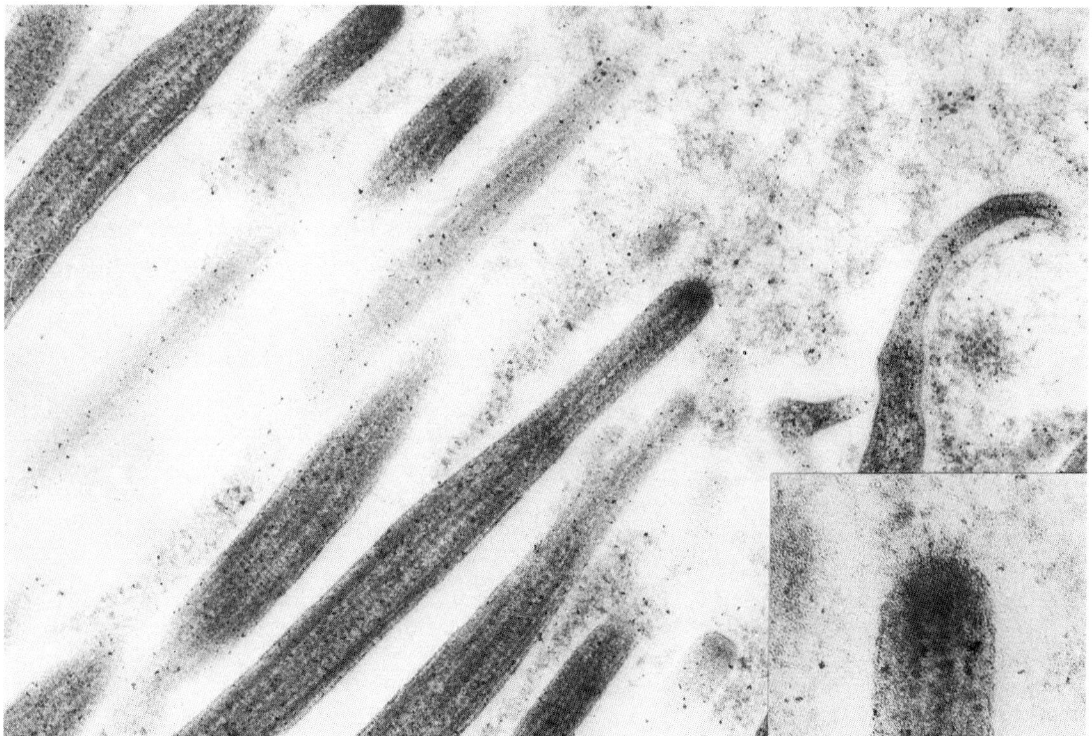

and extend to its tip where they terminate. The complete ciliary beat results from sliding and bending of the adjacent peripheral microtubular doublets across one another.

In recent years, electron microscopy has shown the presence of 5 claw-like projections arising from the apices of the cilia.

The surface area of the bronchial tree is 0.5 m^2. It has been estimated that there are approximately 3×10^{12} cilia in the bronchial mucosa in man. Cilia beat normally at a frequency of 12-14 Hz and provide mucus transport rates of approximately 0.1 cm/min in terminal bronchioles, increasing to about 1 cm/min in the trachea.

Cilia beat in a whip-like fashion consisting of a recovery stroke as they bend backwards through the sol-like periciliary fluid followed by an effector stroke during which the cilium moves forward into an erect position and pushes on the under-surface of the overlying mucus blanket, propelling it towards the larynx. Ciliary beat

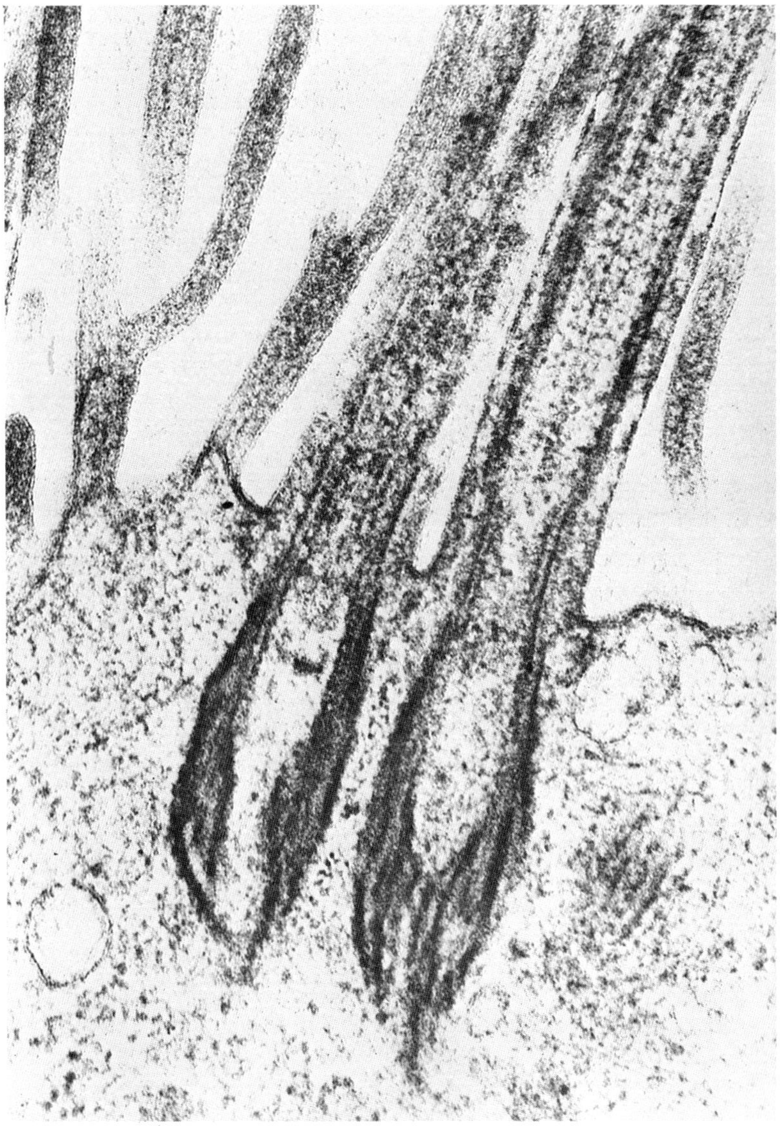

Fig. 11: Cilia showing basal bodies.
Cilia originate in basal bodies (0.5 μm in length), located just beneath the surface of the ciliated cells. Microtubular doublets of the axoneme arise from these basal bodies. The external membrane of the cilia is a direct extension of the cell membrane.

TEM
Magnification: 115,000:1

frequency may be affected by a number of physiological and pathological factors such as temperature or cigarette smoke. At the base of each cilium, the rather dense cytoplasm condenses to form the basal body, an elongated cylindrical structure approximately 0.5 μm in length. The ciliary microtubules together with the other ultrastructural components, which together constitute the axoneme, arise from the basal body. The basal body consists of nine microtubular triplets and two of these tubules continue upwards as the doublets of the axoneme towards the apex of the cilium.

Cilia beat rhythmically in a sequential, co-ordinated manner such that each cilium is slightly out of phase with the one adjacent to it. This results in metachronal waves of ciliary beating which are transmitted to the overlying mucus. In addition to co-ordination of beating within cells, there is also co-ordination of beating between cells of the ciliated epithelium and this produces continuous transport of the mucus blanket towards the pharynx.

Fig. 12: Intercellular desmosome between two bronchial epithelial cells.
Between the cell membranes of two adjacent cells are regularly layered light and dark zones. The inner zone consists of a granular high contrast layer, on either side of which there is a lighter zone. The dense cell membrane borders on a fine filamentous, relatively dense zone in the cytoplasmic matrix.

TEM
Magnification: 68,000:1

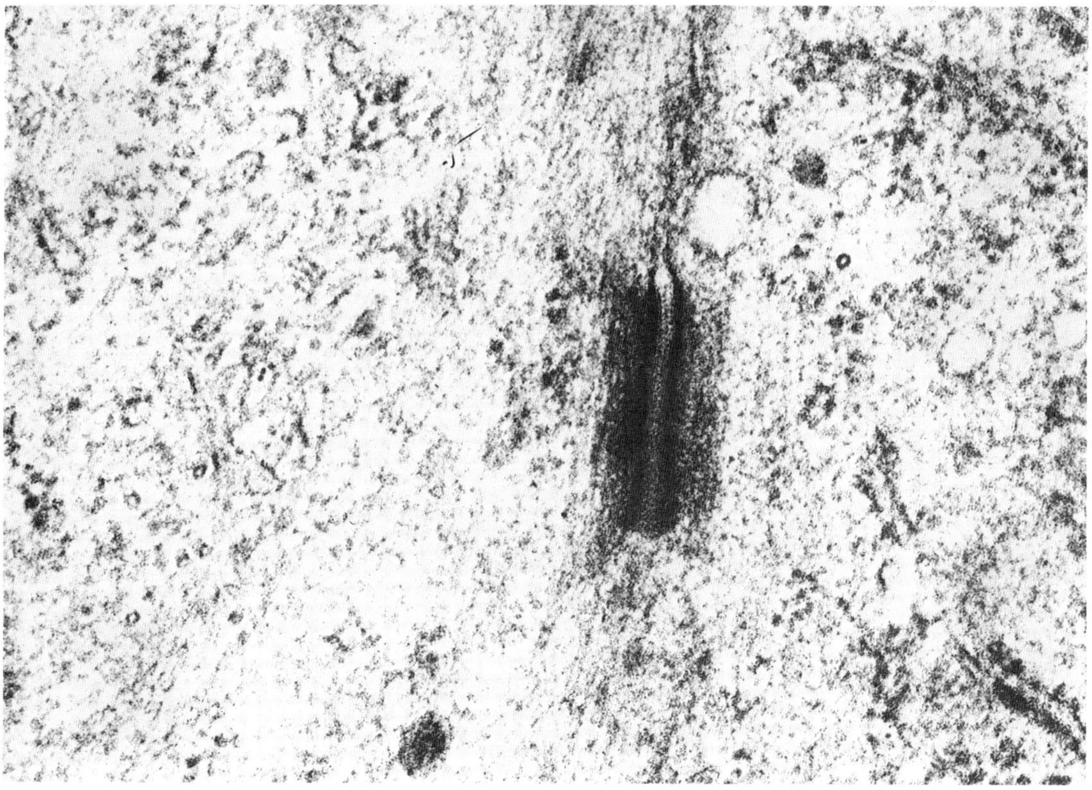

2.3. Goblet Cells

The mucus-producing cells of the respiratory epithelium are called goblet cells because they are shaped like a wine-glass in longitudinal section. The centre of these cells is filled with mucous granules. Airway globlet cells, like those of the gastrointestinal tract, occupy the width of the respiratory epithelium but are narrower and more elongated. Like the ciliated cells, the goblet cells are attached to the basal lamella by slender cytoplasmic extensions that interdigitate between the basal cells.

The ratio of goblet cells to ciliated cells is approximately 1:5 in the trachea, but in more peripheral airways the relative number of goblet cells decreases progressively. In normal man, goblet cells are rare or absent in terminal bronchioles and are not found distal to the terminal bronchiole, except in pathological conditions. Goblet cells are usually seen singly, surrounded by ciliated cells. However, they may also occur in small clusters.

Normally, goblet cells are seen in varying stages of the secretory cycle. During maturation, the secretory granules have a floccular structure that appears increasingly loose towards the cell apex. The granular membranes become progressively thinner and eventually rupture, resulting in a secretory plug. As the secretory granules occupy more of the cytoplasm, the other cytoplasmic structures are displaced towards the periphery and base of the cell.

At maturity, the dome-like lumenal surface of the cell juts approximately 5 μm into the airway lumen, a small hole appears in the cell membrane and the secretion is discharged into the lumen to join the gel phase of the mucous layer, floating above the periciliary fluid and cilia.

Secretions are then transported towards the larynx by mucociliary transport. Following release of the secretions, the cell again becomes a very slender structure which reconstitutes its apical cell membrane and resumes the secretory cycle.

On electron microscopy, the cytoplasm of the goblet cells appears relatively dense. It contains mitochondria and a membranous endoplasmic reticulum, covered with ribosomes. The nucleus is characterized by a dense chromatin network and lies towards the base of the cell. Above the nucleus there is a relatively large Golgi apparatus consisting of a mound of flattened vacuoles surrounded by vesicles. Between the Golgi apparatus and the cell apex, the cell is stuffed with secretory granules, varying in size and electron density.

The cell membrane consists of airway lumen oriented microvilli of varying length that project into the sol-like periciliary fluid. It is postulated that these microvilli function to increase the surface area of the cell membrane. Their function is not certain, but it is thought that they act to secrete or absorb fluid and electrolytes as well as other substances into or from the periciliary fluid. Goblet cells form desmosomes with adjacent cells, which establish intimate contact between their cell membranes. The surrounding cytoplasmic matrix contains a fine filamentous structure directed towards the desmosome.

Fig. 13: Epithelial surface with secretions removed showing the wave-like contour of a cluster of cilia. Dome-shaped goblet cells bulge into the lumen between the cilia.

SEM
Magnification: 10,000:1

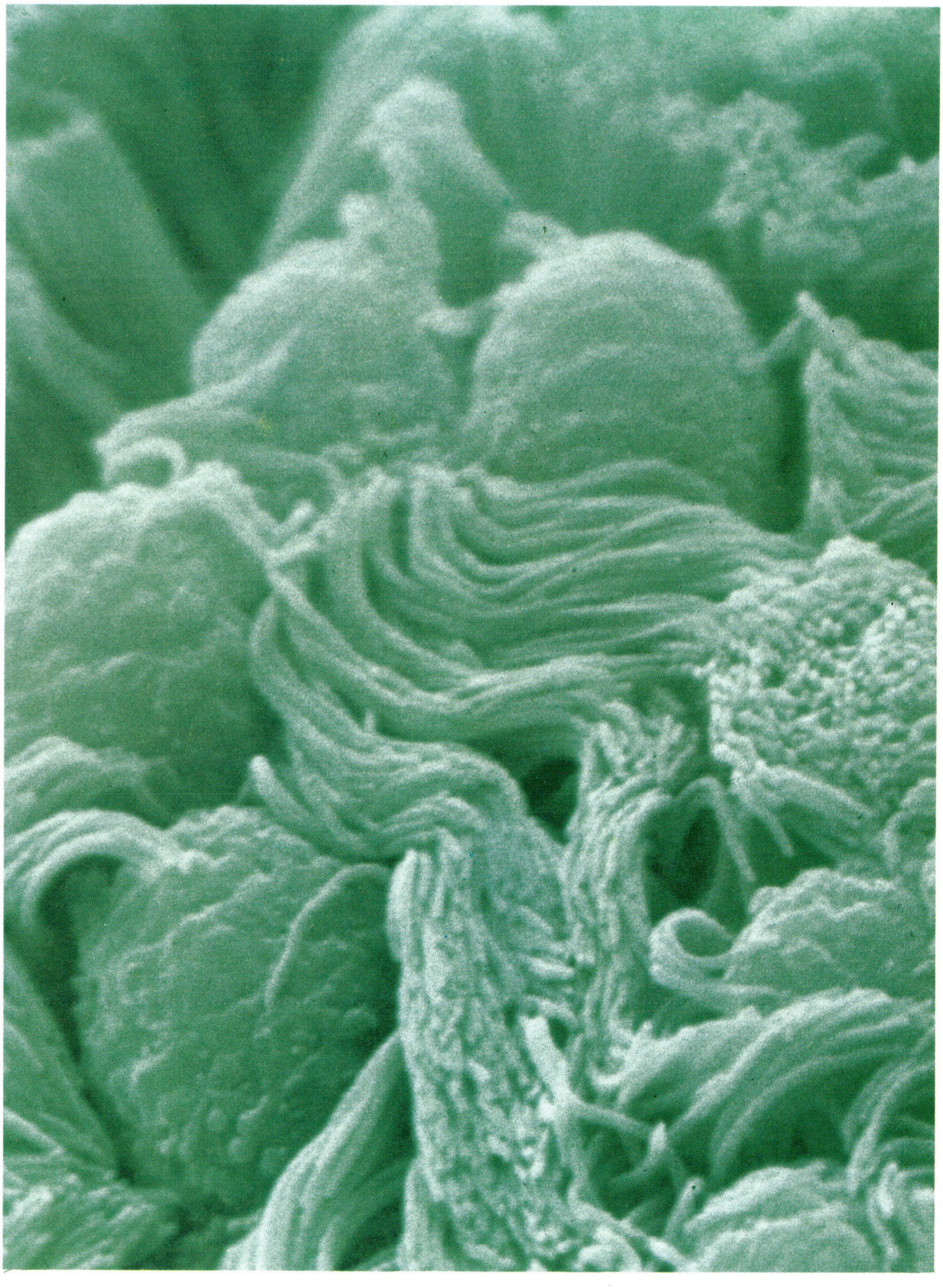

Fig. 14: Secreting goblet cell.

Initially, the secretory granules (Sg) are outlined by limiting membranes. These membranes disappear in the apical portion of the cell and the granules coalesce into larger secretory complexes. Secretions are then ejected in the form of a secretory plug from the funnel-shaped apical cell opening. Cilia are seen on either side of the secretory plug. The secreted material contributes to the gel phase of the mucous blanket at the tips of the cilia.

TEM
Magnification: 13,500:1

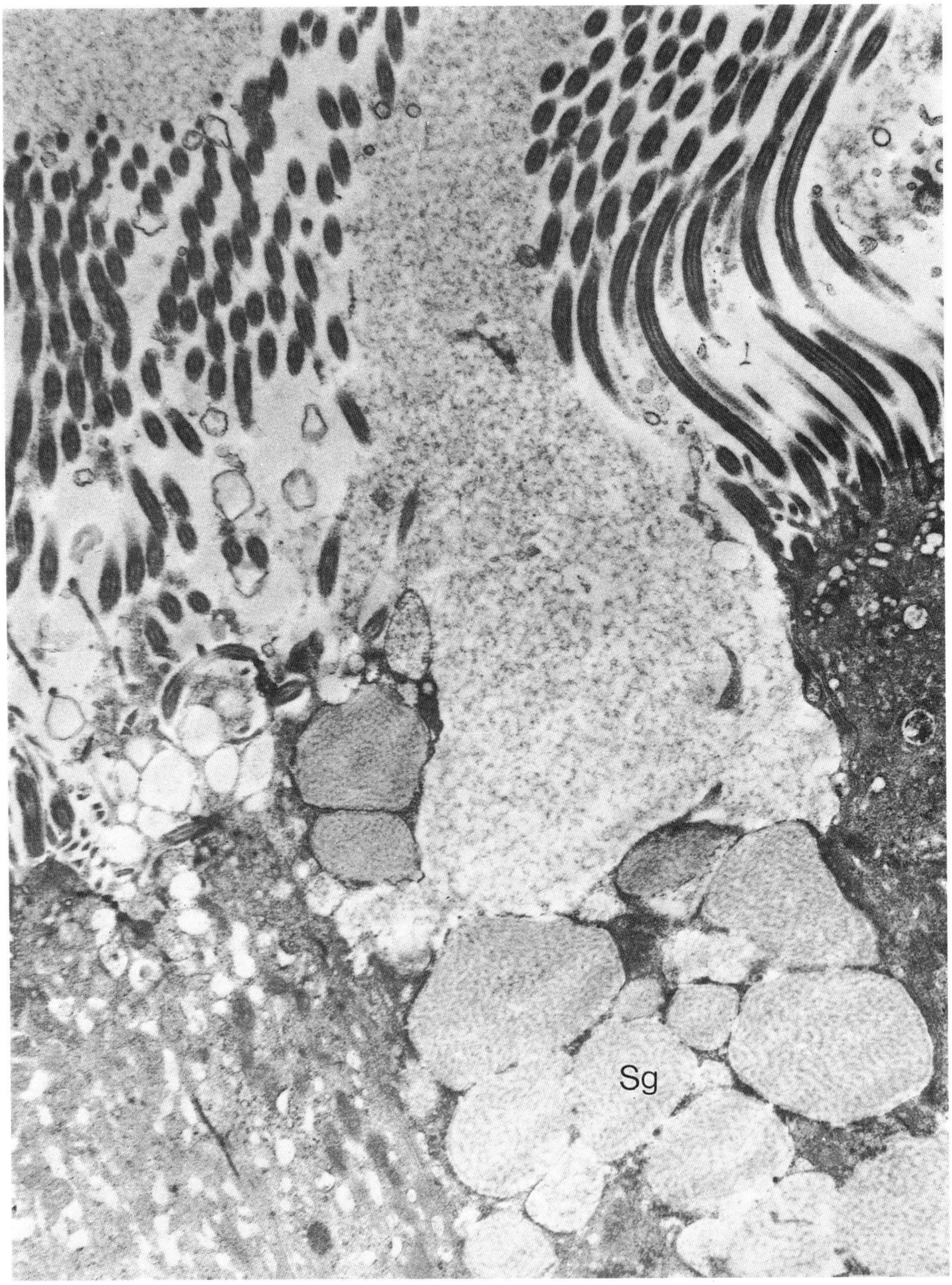

2.4. The Peribronchial Glands

In the human bronchial mucosa, the majority of the mucus is produced by seromucous glands located in the submucosa.

These glands develop as solid epithelial processes after the fourth embryonal month. They are mixed tubuloalveolar glands with seromucous acini which terminate in a common secretory duct. The secretory ducts run obliquely beneath the epithelium and undergo a funnel-like widening just proximal to their orifice. Near the orifice the duct epithelium is ciliated, but more distally it is replaced by a multi-layered cylindrical epithelium, which becomes increasingly flattened to be replaced eventually by an epithelium whose cells are about 70 μm wide and contain numerous mitochondria. Most of the glands are located between the cartilaginous rings and the pars membranacea of the trachea. In more peripheral bronchi, they decrease both in number and size and are no longer present in bronchioles. The glands vary in size from multibranched tree-like structures to glands consisting of only two branches. In the medium sized bronchi, the glands are particularly densely distributed, as much as one gland per mm^2. Mucous and glandular cells are located in specific parts of the glands so that

Fig. 15: Peribronchial glands.
The glandular acini consist of serous and mucous components in approximately equal proportions. The mucous elements consist of epithelial cells having a similar structure to the goblet cells of the surface epithelium. The apical cytoplasmic zones of the serous epithelial cells contain dense secretory granules. Blood vessels are uniformly distributed around the acini.

LM
Semi-thin section
Stain: Basic fuchsin and methylene blue
Magnification: 1,200:1

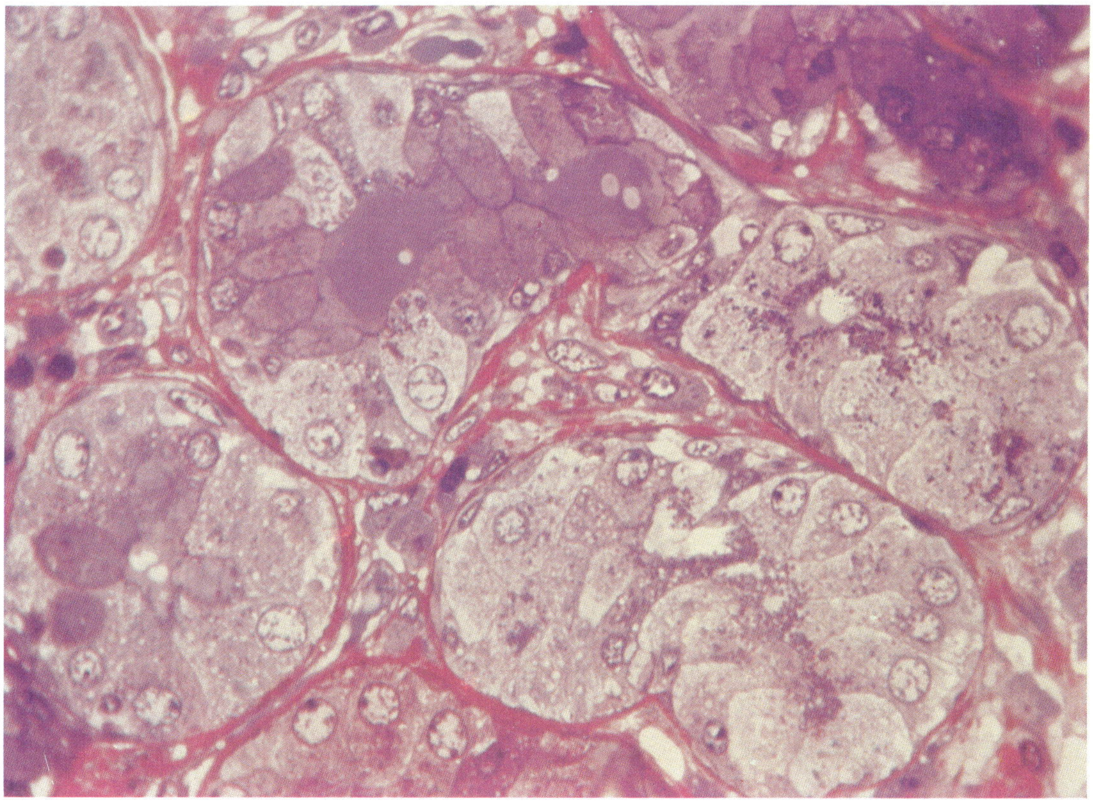

serous secretions usually flow over the mucous cells before reaching the secretory duct. Both the serous and mucous cells of these glands are under autonomic control. The cytoplasm of the glands cannot be transformed directly into secretory granules, hence synthesis of the secretory components occurs in stages which depend on specific intracellular structures.

As a result of enzymatic action on the appropriate substrates, the glandular cells continually produce secretions. Initially there is assembly of the necessary building blocks, such as amino acids, phosphates, etc. Subsequently, intracellular enzyme synthesis occurs, followed by outpouring of secretion. Following a resting phase, the glandular cells are again able to begin absorbing substrates from the blood. As a result of enzyme-protein synthesis, secretory granules are produced which accumulate at the apex of the cell in the middle of the Golgi apparatus. The secretory granules in the serous glandular acini contain, in part, radiodense inner structures, close to a delicate limiting membrane or accumulations of an opaque homogeneous substance. Usually, the secretory granules are excreted into the glandular duct lumen by means of a canal lock-like mechanism. Thus, the apical membranes of the granules fuse with the adjacent cell membrane. These then rupture, releasing the granules, and the basal portions of the granular membranes become the new cell surface membrane. Cellular

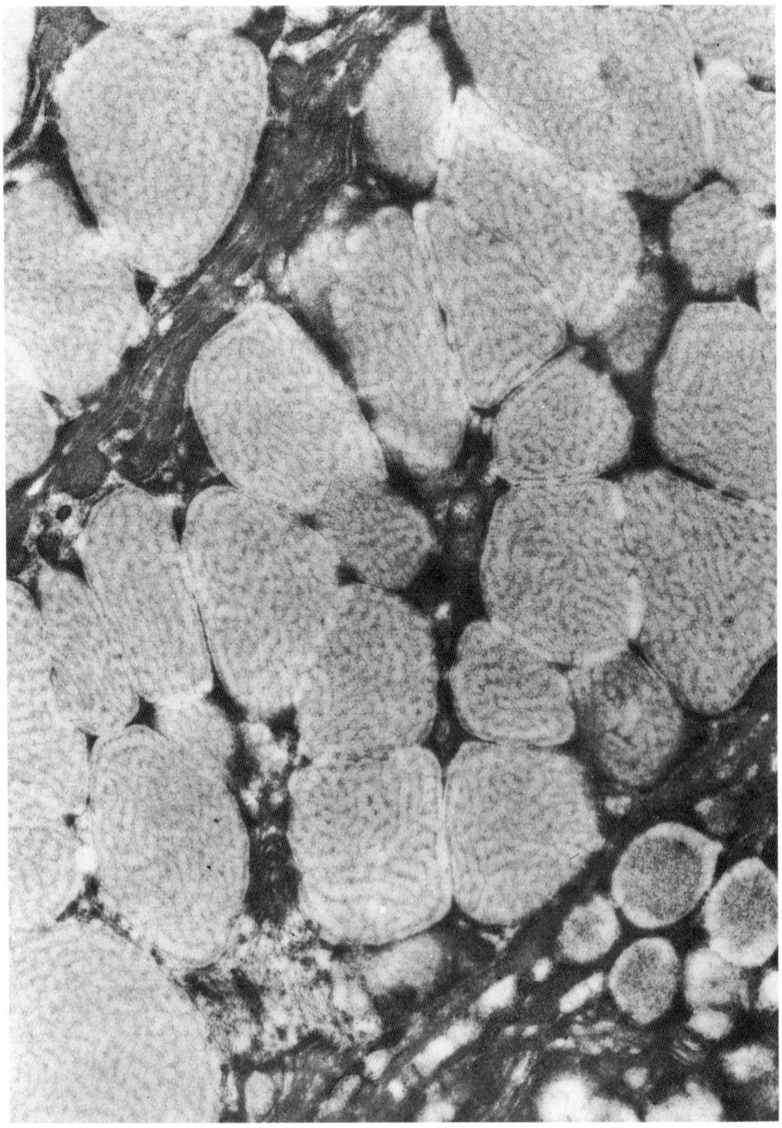

Fig. 16: Secretory granules in the cytoplasm of mucous gland cells in a peribronchial gland. Individual secretory droplets are surrounded by a cytoplasmic membrane. Within the secretory granules lies a filamentous matrix. Between the densely packed secretory granules are strands of endoplasmic reticulum.

TEM
Magnification: 12,500:1

metabolism is probably potentiated by the increased surface area resulting from microvilli at the cell apex and invaginations of the base of the cells.

The mucous components of the peribronchial glands consist of goblet cells containing a basally located nucleus and cytoplasm filled with pre-secretory granules which become confluent towards the cell apex and form large secretory complexes. They are supplied with organelles similar to those of the goblet cells of the surface epithelium. Between the basal cell membrane of the glandular cells and the basal lamella of the acinus lie evenly distributed myoepithelial cells. These cells have a fine fibrillar cytoplasmic structure and lie adjacent to the glandular cells without any associated sarcolemma. It is thought that the myoepithelial cells contract, expressing secretion from the glandular cells.

At electron microsopy, the goblet cells show a clearly polar structure. The usually oval nucleus is located in the basal portions of the cell. The cytoplasm is relatively electron dense and contains mitochondria and membranes of the endoplasmic reticulum with their associated ribosomes. Above the nucleus lies the extensive Golgi apparatus consisting of a pile of flattened saccules surrounded by vesicles.

Above the Golgi apparatus are secretory granules of varying size and electron density. The goblet cells are found in various stages of activity or maturity. Immature goblet cells contain only partly formed secretory granules which do not completely fill the cytoplasm. On the surface of the goblet cells are microvilli of various lenghts. Except when it is actively secreting, the goblet cell surface is continous with the surface of the adjacent ciliated cells. However, at the time of discharge, goblet cells protrude several millimeters into the bronchial lumen pushing aside the adjacent ciliated cells. In this way, the continuity of the ciliated bronchial surface is interrupted only during active secretion. The formation of secretions starts with the separation of electron dense vesicles from the flat Golgi sacs. These pre-secretory granules migrate towards the apical portions of the cell, where with increasing swelling and flocculation, maturation of the mucus occurs. The secretory granules enlarge and become confluent forming large secretory complexes. At the same time, the relative amount of cytoplasm between the secretory components becomes decreased, resulting in the development of larger secretory complexes in the upper portions of the cell. Subsequently, the mucus globules are discharged across the surface of the epithelial cells and into the lumen. Thus, the contents of the apical portion of the cell join the gel phase of the secretory layer, which lies at the tips of the erect cilia, above the periciliary fluid.

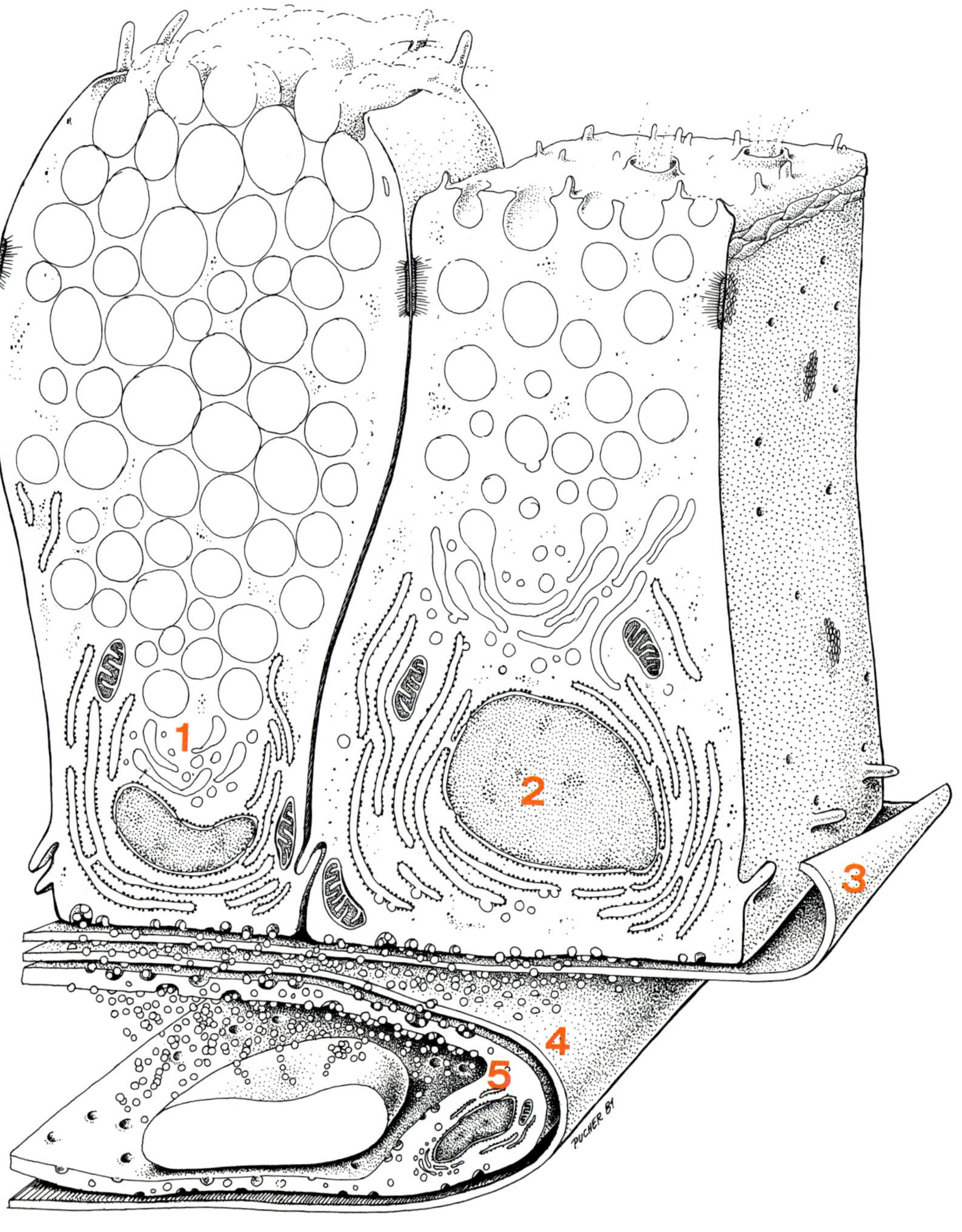

Fig. 17: Three dimensional diagram showing formation of secretions in the glands of the bronchial tree.

1: mucous cell
2: serous cell
3: basal lamella of the glandular epithelium
4: basal lamella of the adjacent capillary
5: capillary showing erythrocyte in cross section

The building blocks from which the secretions are formed reach the epithelial cells from the capillaries by passing through the capillary wall, interstitial space and basal lamella. The organelles of the epithelial cells in the Golgi apparatus and endoplasmic reticulum transform the basic metabolic products into secretory granules, which first appear in the cytoplasm as pro-secretory granules. In the mucous epithelial cells, the secretory granules become confluent to form larger complexes which are then ejected as clumps of mucus. In the serous glandular cells, droplets of secretion fuse with the cell surface individually, thus secretory droplets are secreted by exocytosis onto the epithelial surface.

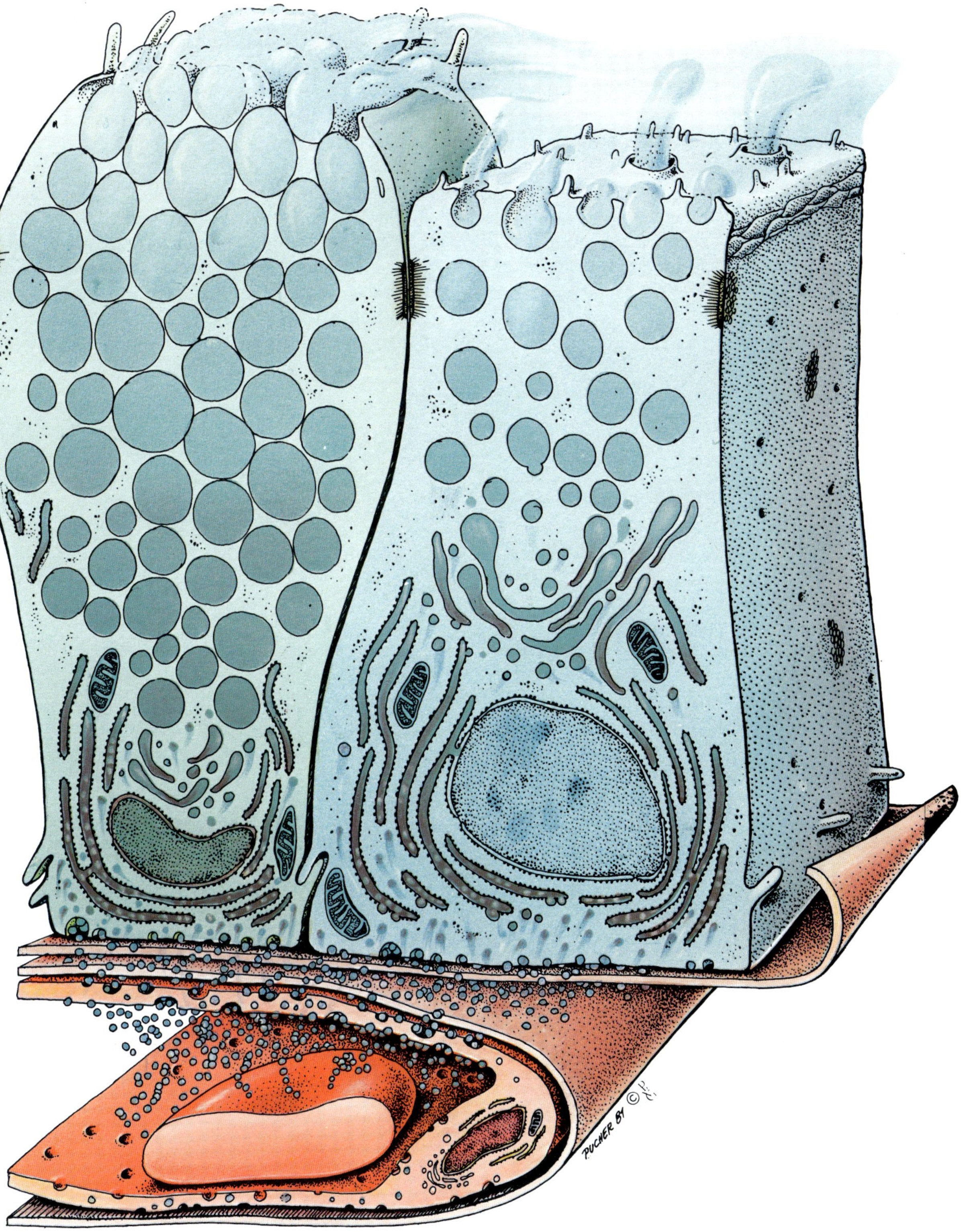

2.5. The Secretory Layer

The secretion covering the bronchial epithelium consists of two layers: a thin watery, sol-like layer about 5-6 μm thick, in which the cilia beat, and above which floats a 2-3 μm gel-like mucus "blanket". The cilia beat rapidly in the sol phase with a very complex bending motion consisting of an effector stroke during which the tip of the erect cilium interacts with the undersurface of the gel layer, followed by a whip-like recovery stroke during which the cilium moves rapidly forwards in the direction of fluid movement and then bends backwards through the periciliary layer before beginning another beat cycle. In this way an escalator-like transport of secretion is accomplished, clearing the airways of inhaled biological and non-biological particles trapped in the mucus.

It is postulated that between the mucous blanket and the periciliary fluid, there is a layer of surfactant, derived from type II alveolar cells, which is also transported mouthwards. Recent morphological findings suggest that the surfactant occupies a narrow, foamy zone consisting of small vesicles, which serves to regulate the surface tension between the sol and gel phases of the airway secretions. Recently, numerous mast cells have been described floating in the bronchial mucus. Their role is not certain, but under normal conditions, by variably releasing mediators, they may function to control the depth of the periciliary fluid, while in asthma, sensitized lumenal mast cells may suddenly release large amounts of mediators of the allergic reaction as a result of rapid degranulation, thus amplifying the resulting inflammatory, bronchospastic and secretory response.

Fig. 18: Mucous layer on the bronchial epithelial surface.
The bronchial mucosa is covered by a layer of mucus (1). This is an important component of the bronchial defence system. The mucous blanket is continually transported from the periphery towards the larynx by rapidly beating cilia. The cilia beat in the low viscosity, periciliary fluid clearly seen between the mucous blanket and the lumenal surface of the ciliated cell (2). Note that the cilia do not enter the denser mucous layer during the beat cycle.

TEM
Magnification: 2,400:1

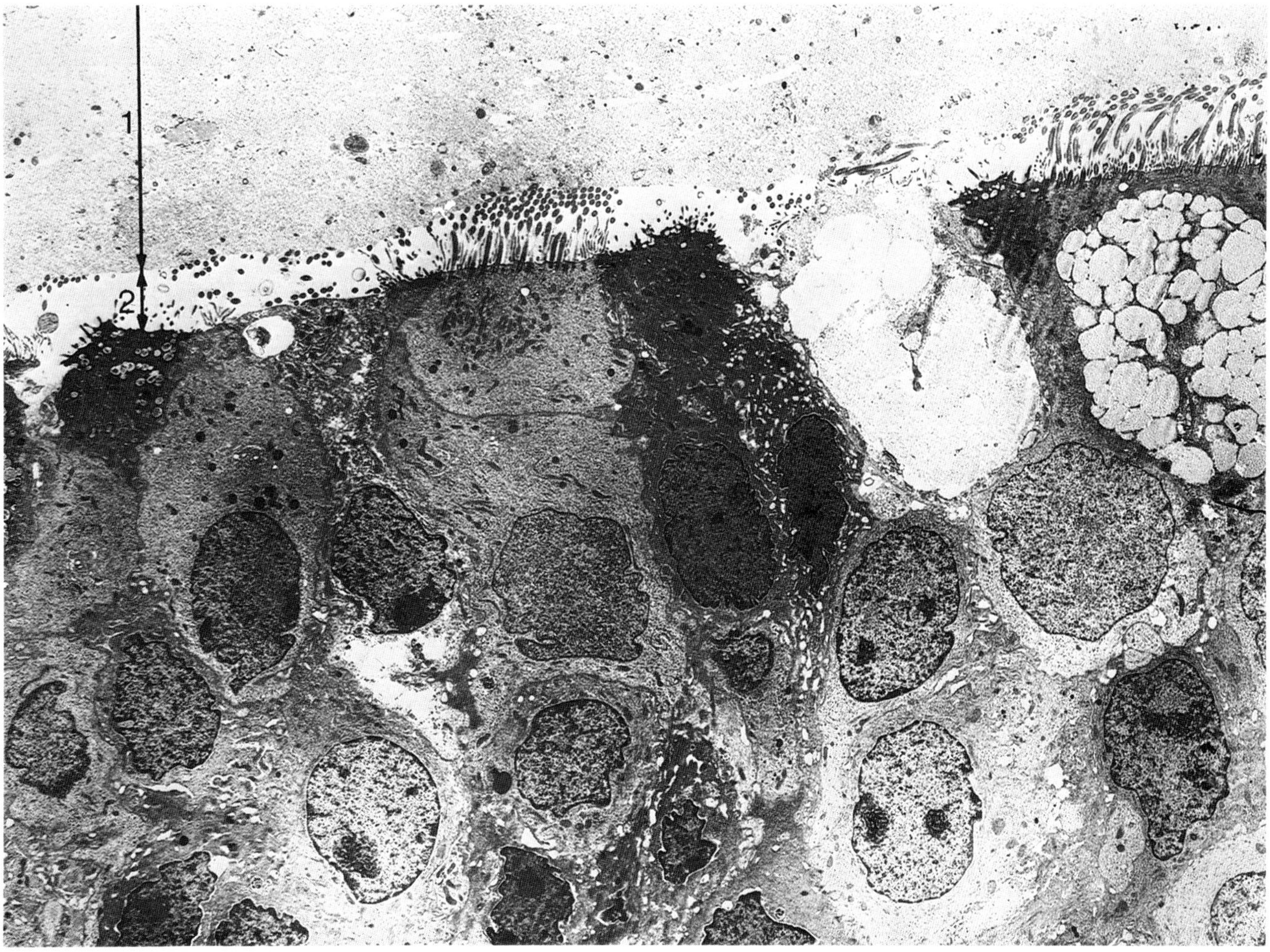

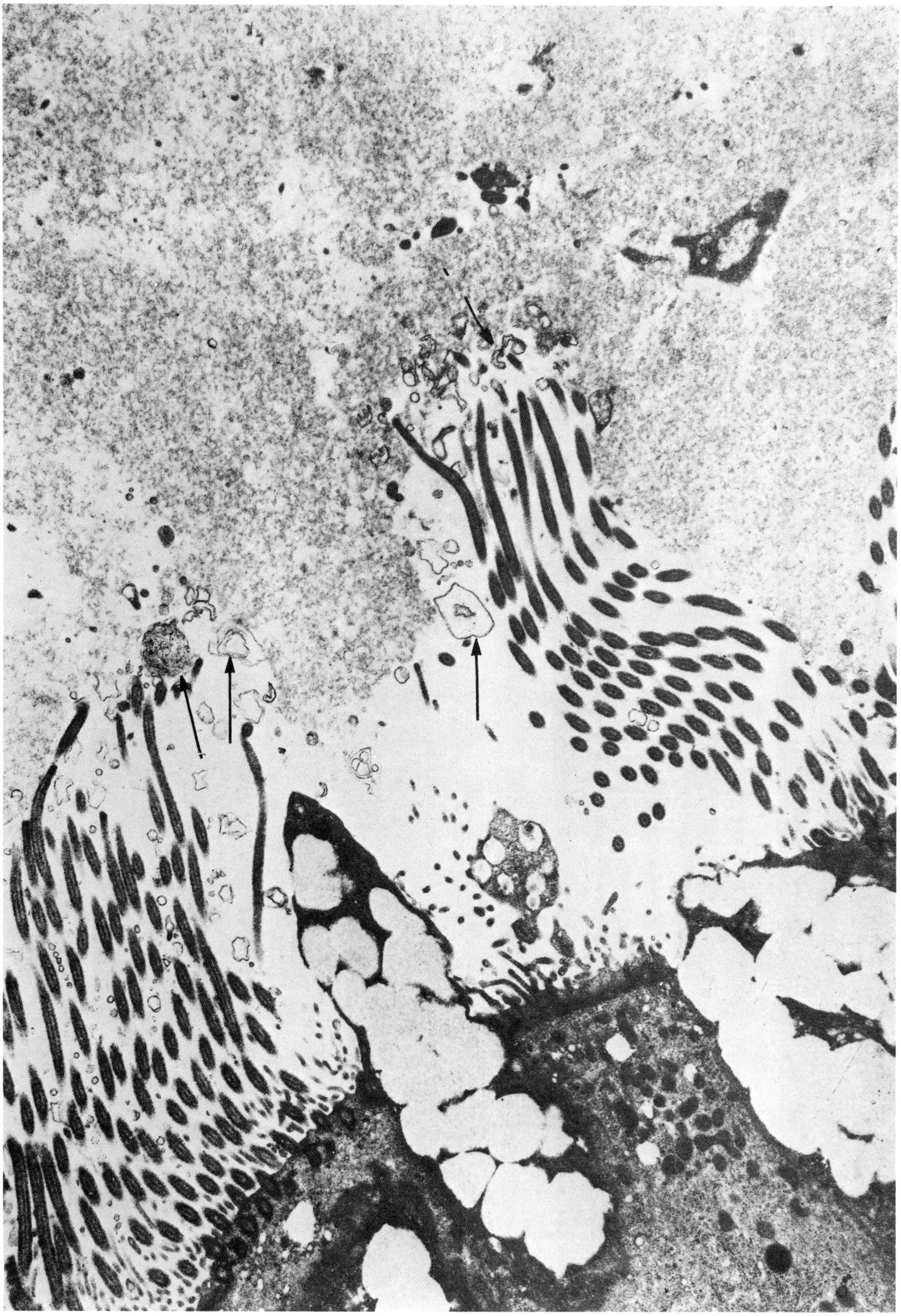

←

Fig. 19: Mucus transport.
Normal mucus transport is accomplished by the rapid beating of cilia in the low viscosity, watery, periciliary fluid (clear zone) and interaction with the gel-like mucous layer (granular zone). In the periciliary fluid are vesicular structures (arrows) surrounded by a limiting phospholipid membrane (surfactant). Microvilli, much smaller sometimes branching projections, cover the surface of the ciliated cell and lie between the cilia.

TEM
Magnification: 9,500:1

Alveolar Section

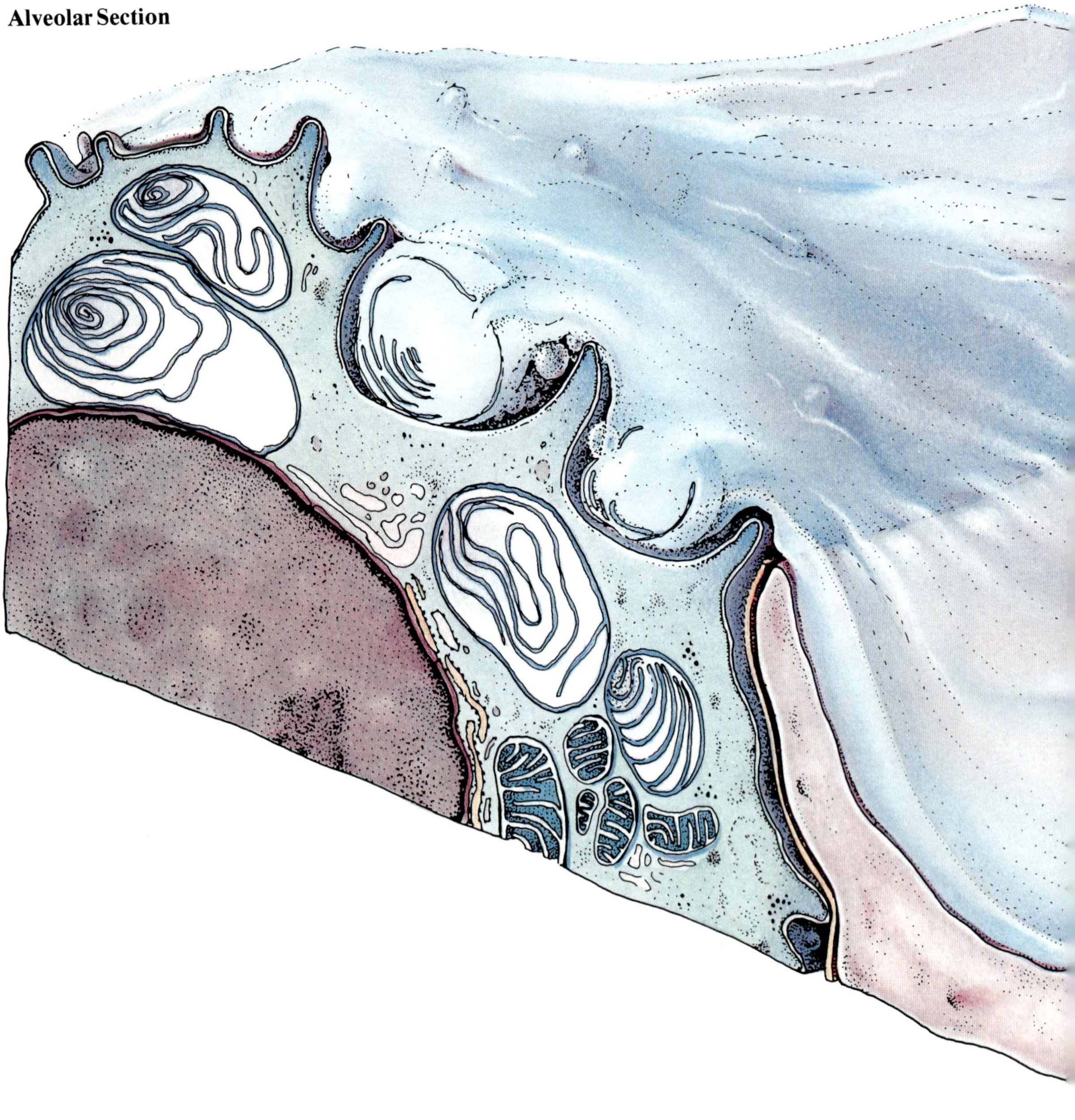

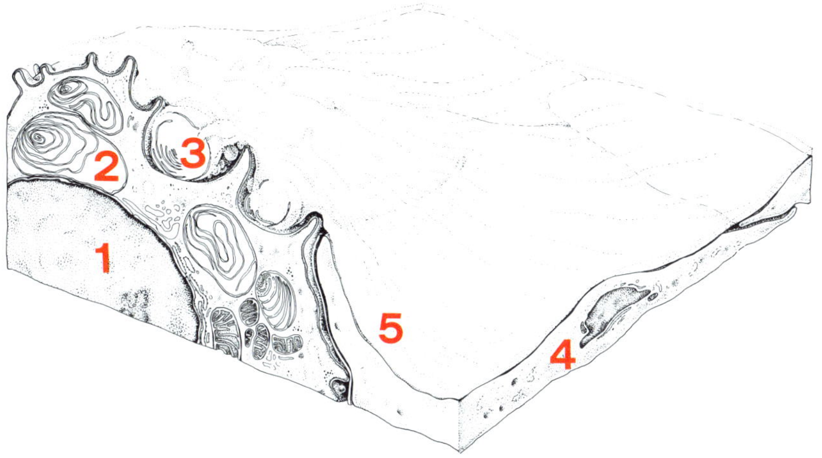

Fig. 20: Diagram of pneumocyte II: Storage and release of surfactant.
1: nucleus of pneumocyte II
2: lamellar body of pneumocyte II
3: excretion of surfactant
4: pneumocyte I
5: surfactant layer consisting of a watery phase and a contrast-rich phospholipid layer which smooths the surface of the alveolar wall.

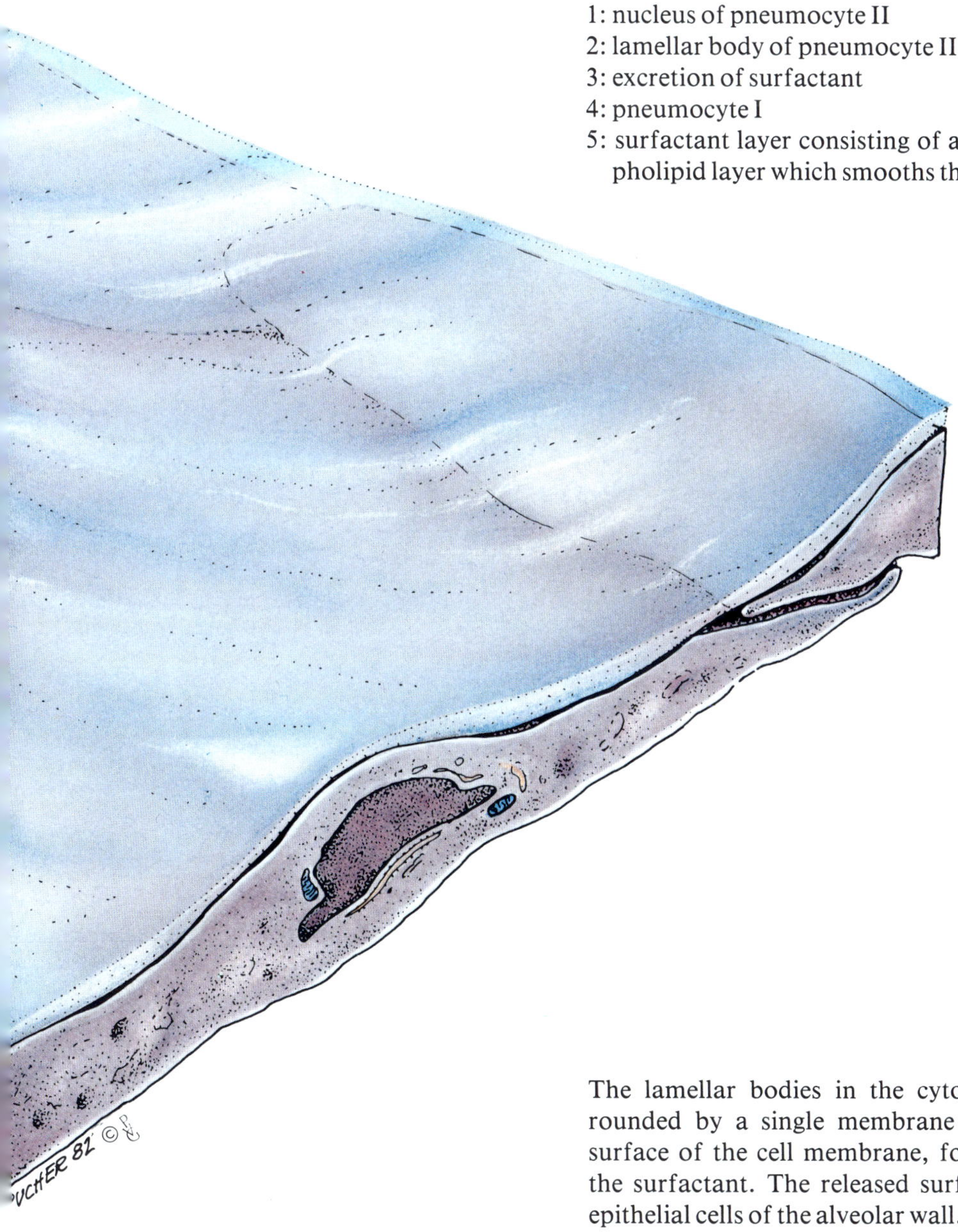

The lamellar bodies in the cytoplasm of the pneumocyte II are surrounded by a single membrane which becomes attached to the inner surface of the cell membrane, following which the cell opens to release the surfactant. The released surfactant spreads over the surface of the epithelial cells of the alveolar wall.

Fig. 21a: Transitional zone from alveolar to bronchial system.
Around the alveolar duct are epithelial lined alveoli. The cell boundaries of the epithelial cells can be identified because of slight depressions in the surface of the epithelium. The terminal bronchiole originates from the alveolar duct. The terminal bronchiole can be readily identified by the numerous dome-shaped secretory caps of Clara cells on its surface. Immediately adjacent to the alveolar ducts, there are no ciliated cells in the terminal bronchiole.

SEM
Magnification: 800:1

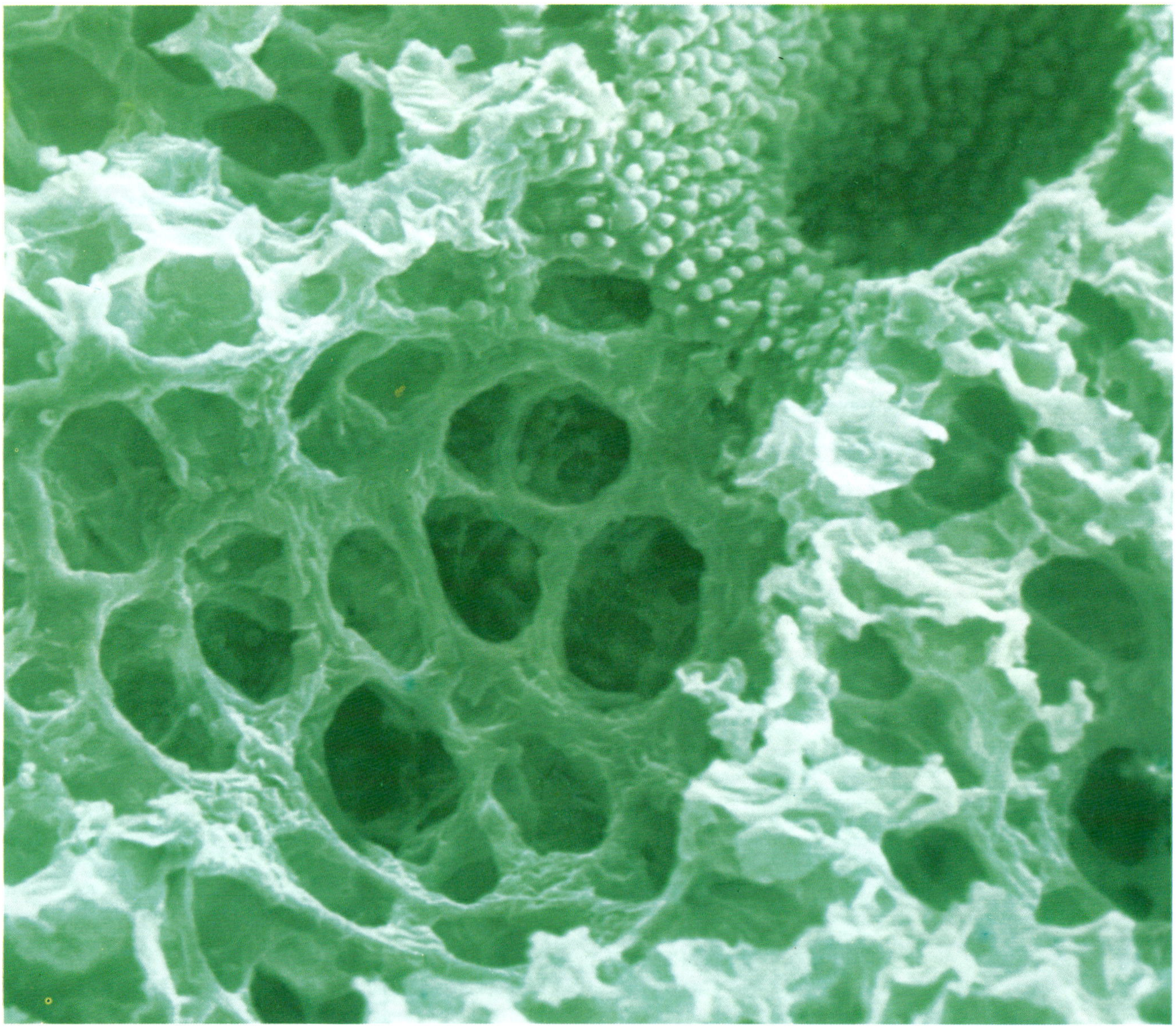

Fig. 21b: Foamy surface active material between tangentially sectioned cilia in the sol phase of the secretory layer. This material is in part contained within individual osmiophilic membranes. These consist of delicate layered membranous structures similar to those representing the stored form of surfactant in the pneumocyte II. The thickness of the membranes corresponds to that of the osmiophilic phase of the surfactant layer in the alveoli.

TEM
Magnification: 42,000:1

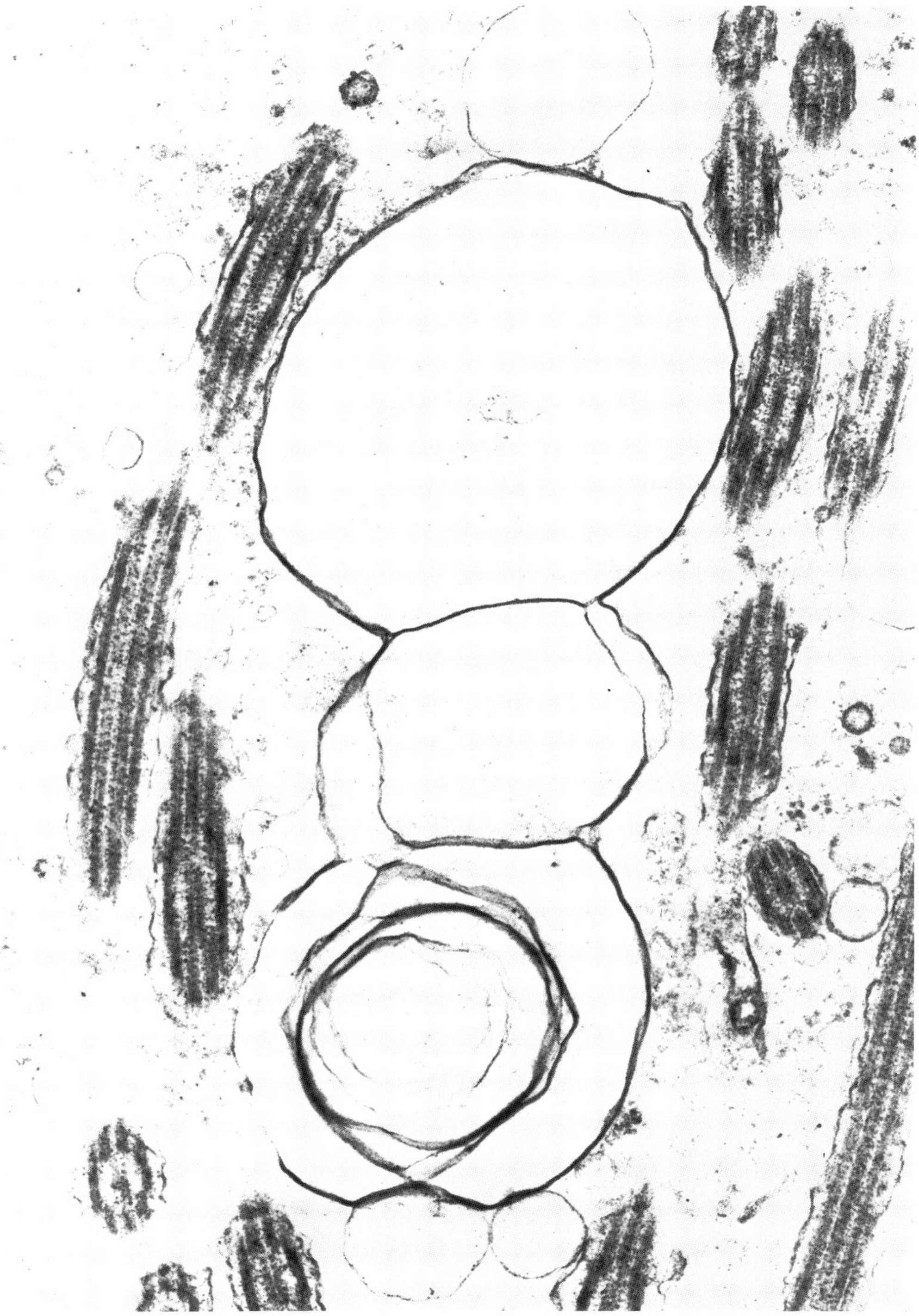

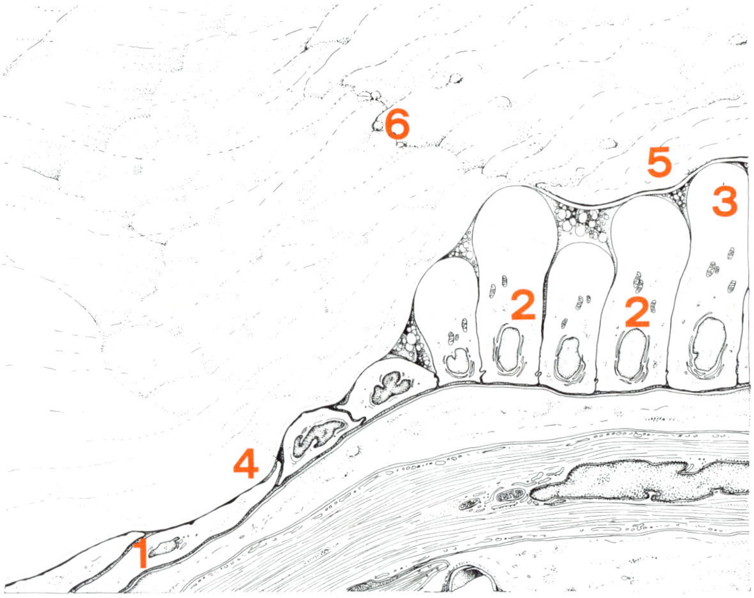

Fig. 22: Transition zone between the alveolar system and terminal bronchiole and between the surfactant and mucous layer.

1: pneumocyte I lining the alveolar wall
2: Clara cells of the terminal bronchiole
3: secretory caps of Clara cells on epithelial surface
4: surfactant layer covering alveoli and alveolar duct
5: secretory layer on the surface of the bronchiolar mucosa
6: transition zone between surfactant layer and secretory layer with transformation of surfactant into vesicular structures.

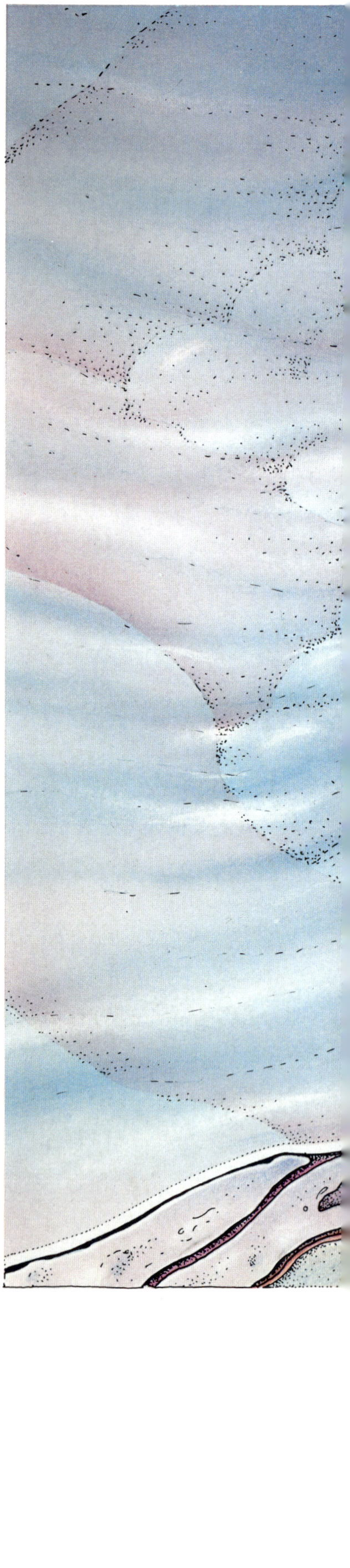

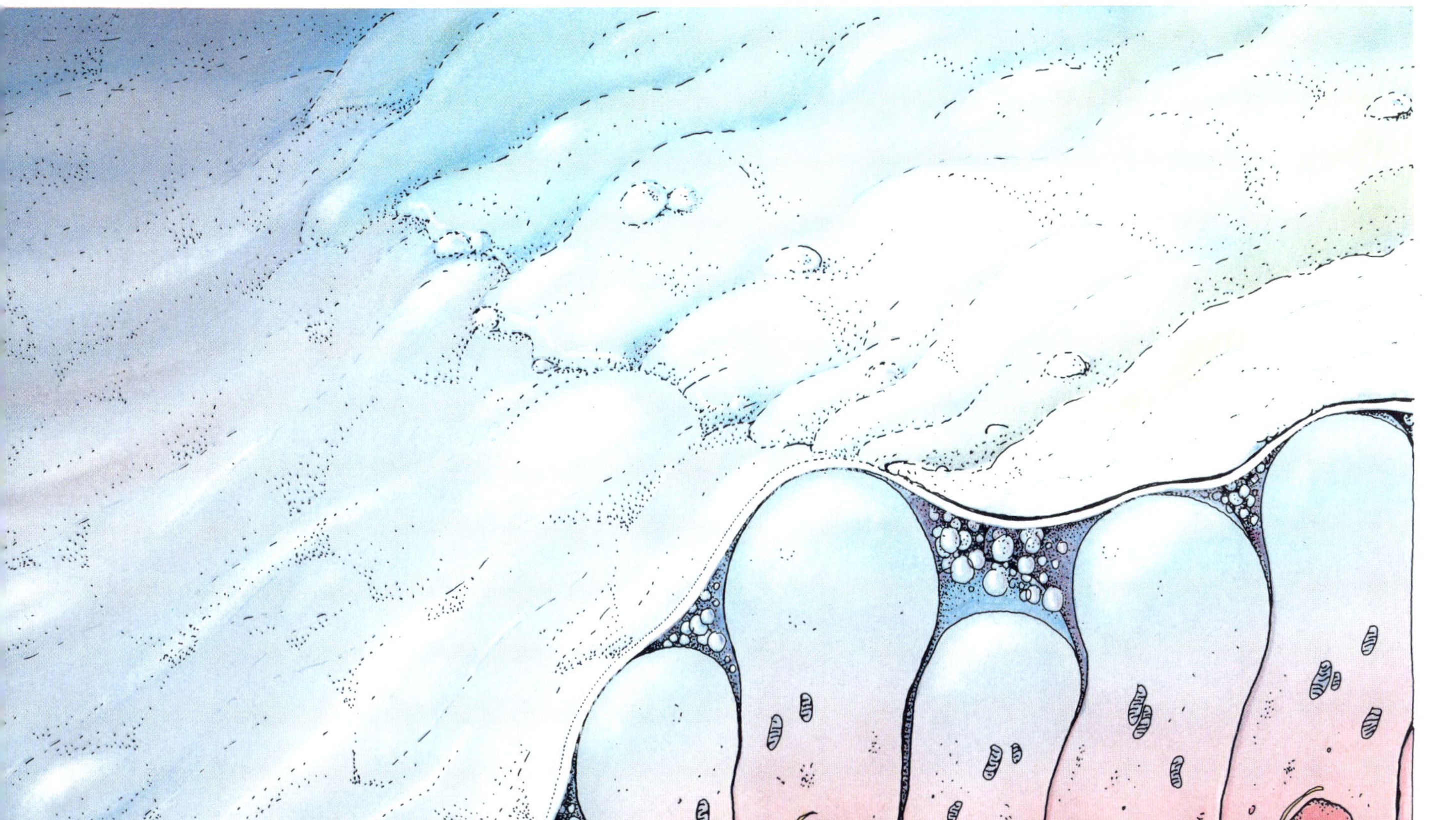

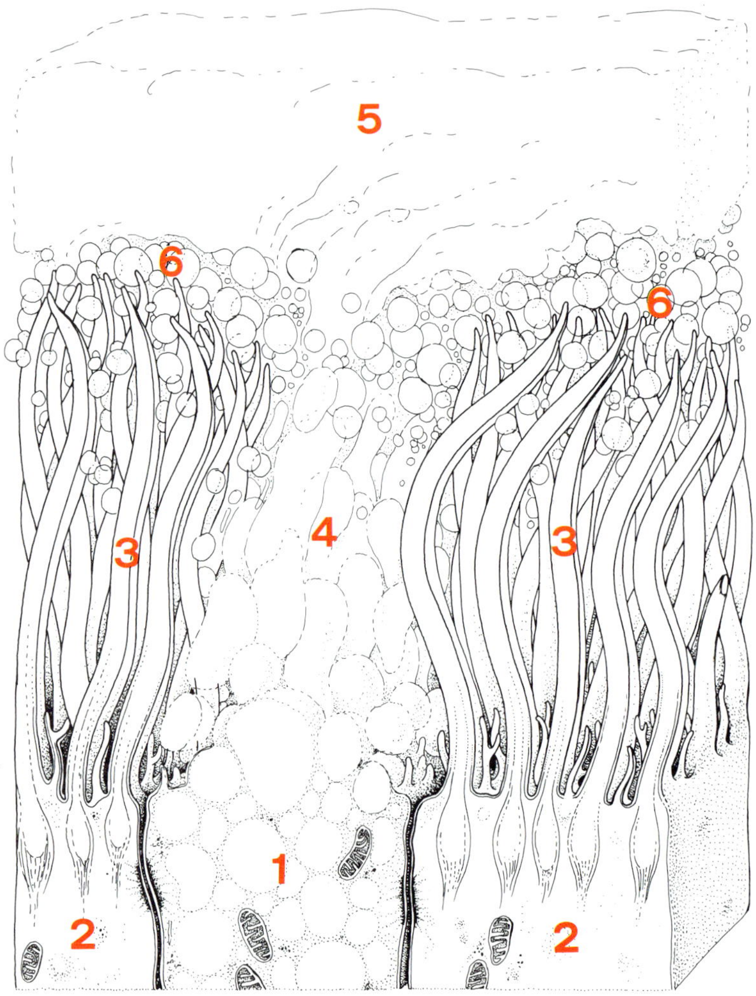

Fig. 23: Bronchial mucosa surface showing the arrangement of secretory layer.

1: secreting goblet cell
2: ciliated cell
3: cilia beating in the sol phase of the secretory layer
4: secretory portion of the goblet cell between the cilia and immediately adjacent to the cell surface. Droplets of secretion are delineated by membrane remnants
5: gel phase of secretory layer
6: surfactant material indicated as a foamy layer consisting of vesicular structures in the transitional zone between the sol and gel phase of the secretory layer

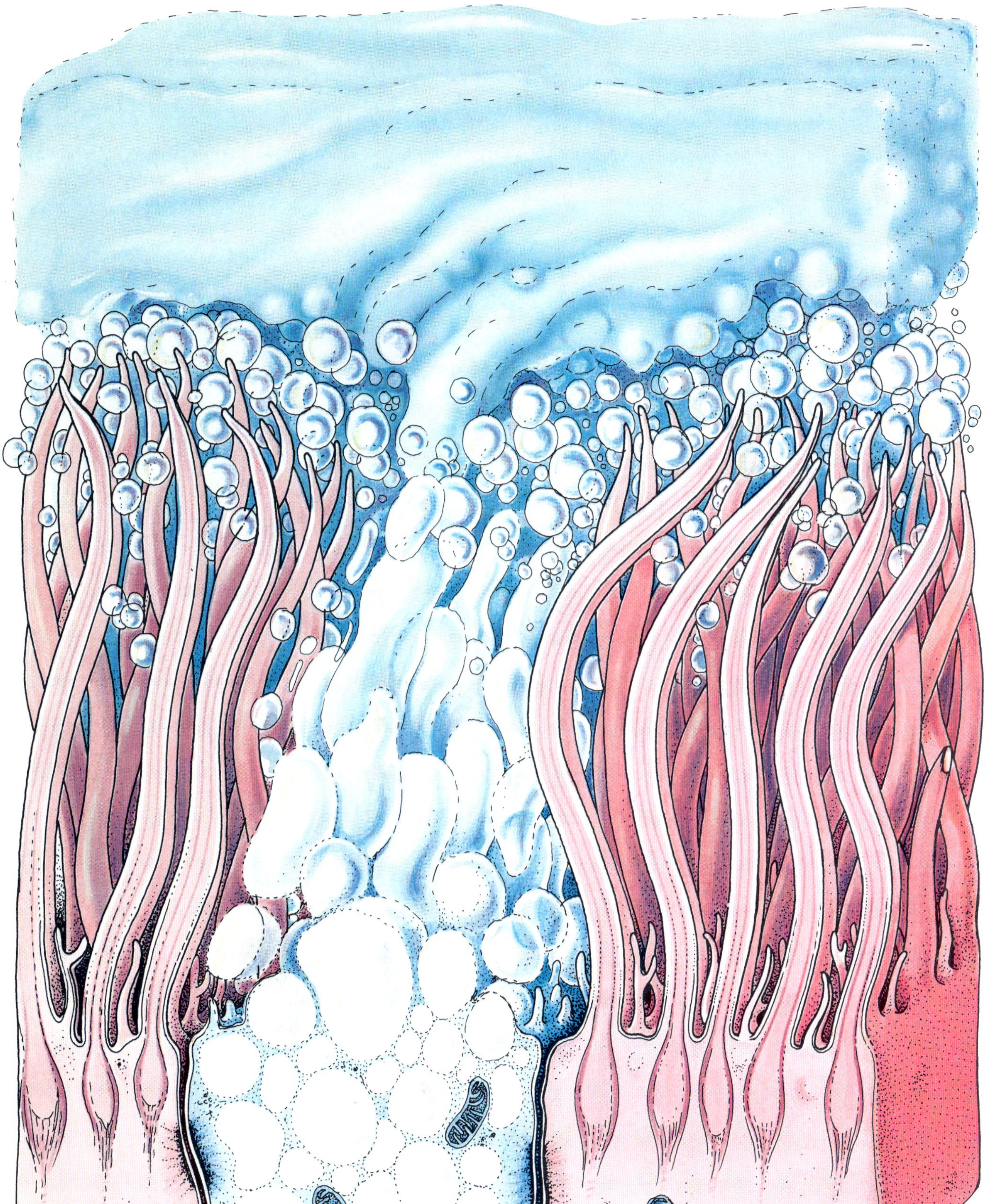
PUCHER 82 ©

2.6. Immunocomptent Cells in the Stroma of the Bronchial Epithelium

Cells in the lamina propria of the bronchial mucosa produce immunoglobulins which enter the airway secretions. Thus, the mucus and mucosa of the respiratory tract form a major defence against inhaled pathogenic organisms. Immunological reactions play an important part in these defence mechanisms. In general, the respiratory tract may participate in all immunological reactions. The airways may participate in immuno-pathological responses of an antigen-antibody reaction initiated elsewhere, or alternatively, immune reactions may occur locally in the lung with little, if any, effect on other organs.

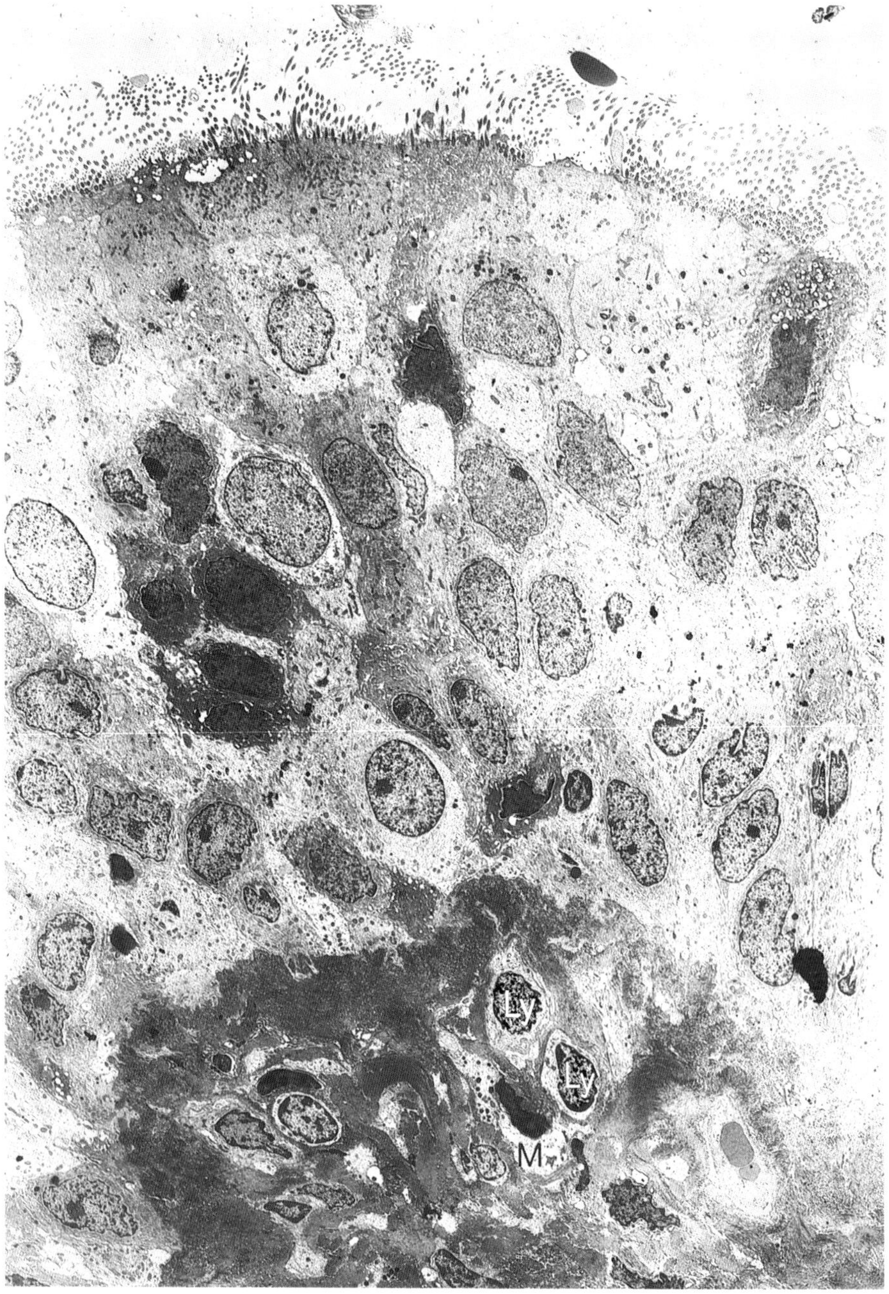

Fig. 24: Bronchial mucosa. Immunocompetent cells in the subepithelial layer of connective tissue: lymphovytes (Ly) and mast cells (M).

TEM
Magnification: 1,800:1

In the bronchial mucosa, reactions centering on molecular antibodies predominate. Immunoglobulin A (IgA), particularly secretory - IgA, plays an important role in mucosal defences. S-IgA in the mucus performs a frontline immunological function in that it combines with pathogenic agents, causes their agglutination and prevents them from becoming established in the bronchial mucosa. In the type I reaction, mast cells are particularly important. They are located mainly in the subepithelial connective tissue throughout the respiratory tract, particularly in relation to submucosal blood vessels and they may pass into the bronchial epithelium through the basal lamella. Mast cells contain numerous cytoplasmic granules which store mediators that may be released during immunological reactions and account for immediate (type I) hypersensitivity.

Fig. 25: Mast cell with collagen fibrils.
These cells contain evenly distributed, high density granules containing mediators throughout the cytoplasm. On the cell surface there are fine projections. The mast cell granules show a typical whorled lamellar ultrastructure (inset).

TEM
Magnification: 18,000:1
Magnification (inset): 56,000:1

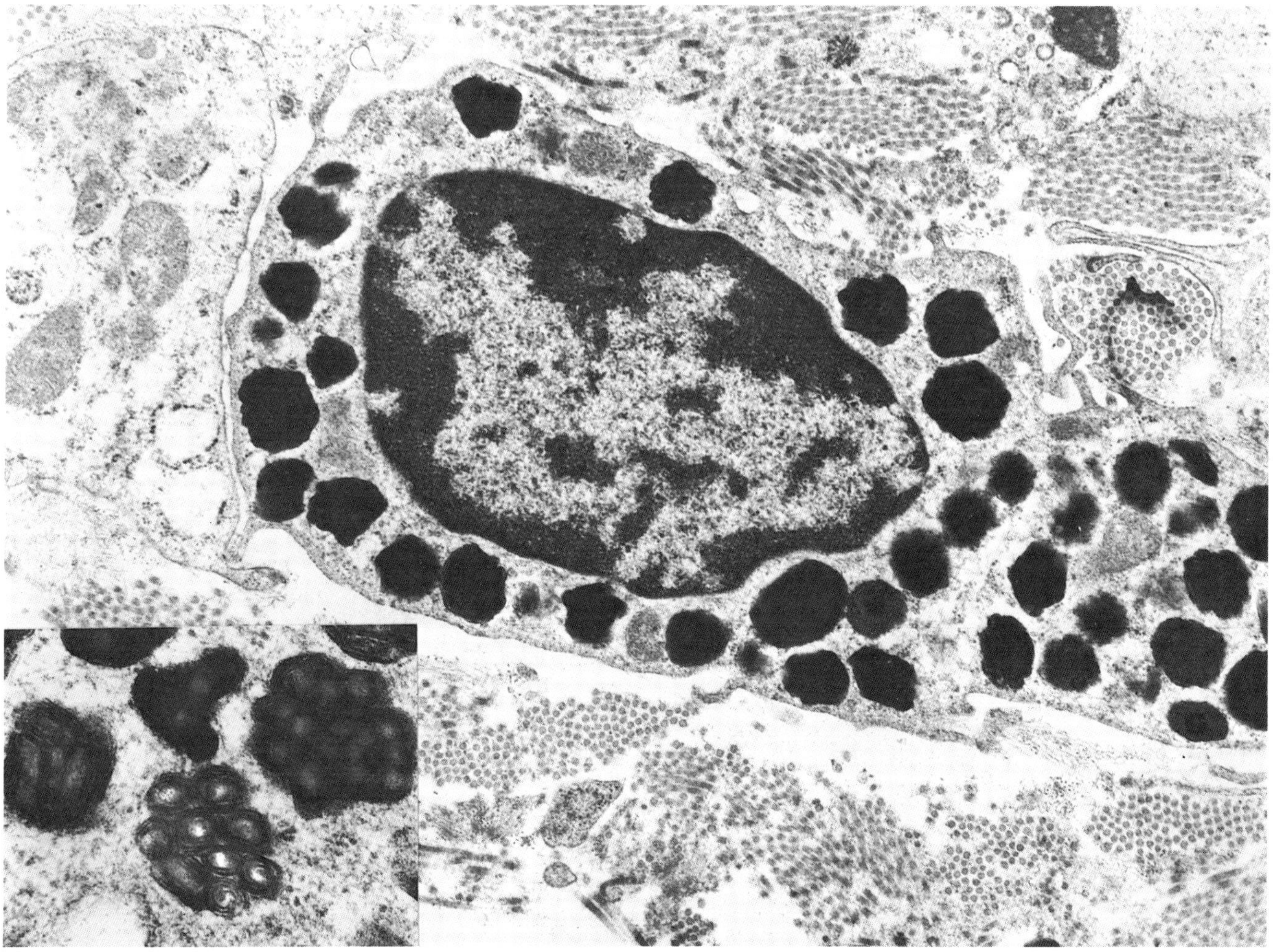

Figs. 26a, b: Intraepithelial mast cell.
Mast cells (M) can penetrate the surface epithelium of the bronchial mucosa. The intracellular junctions between epithelial cells open and mast cells push cytoplasmic projections of varying thickness between the epithelial cells until they reach the epithelial surface.

TEM
Magnification a: 2,400:1
b: 8,500:1

b:

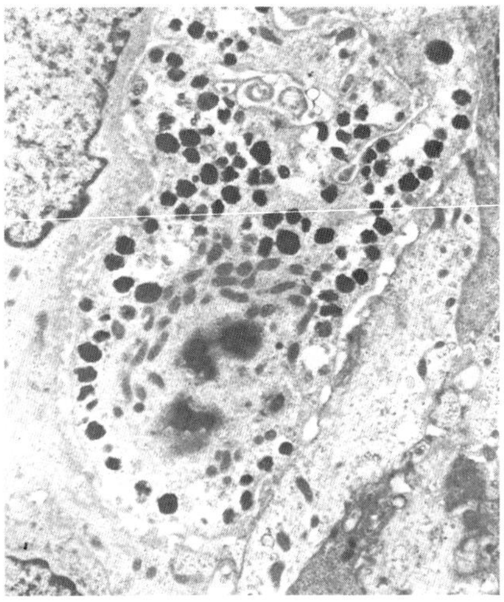

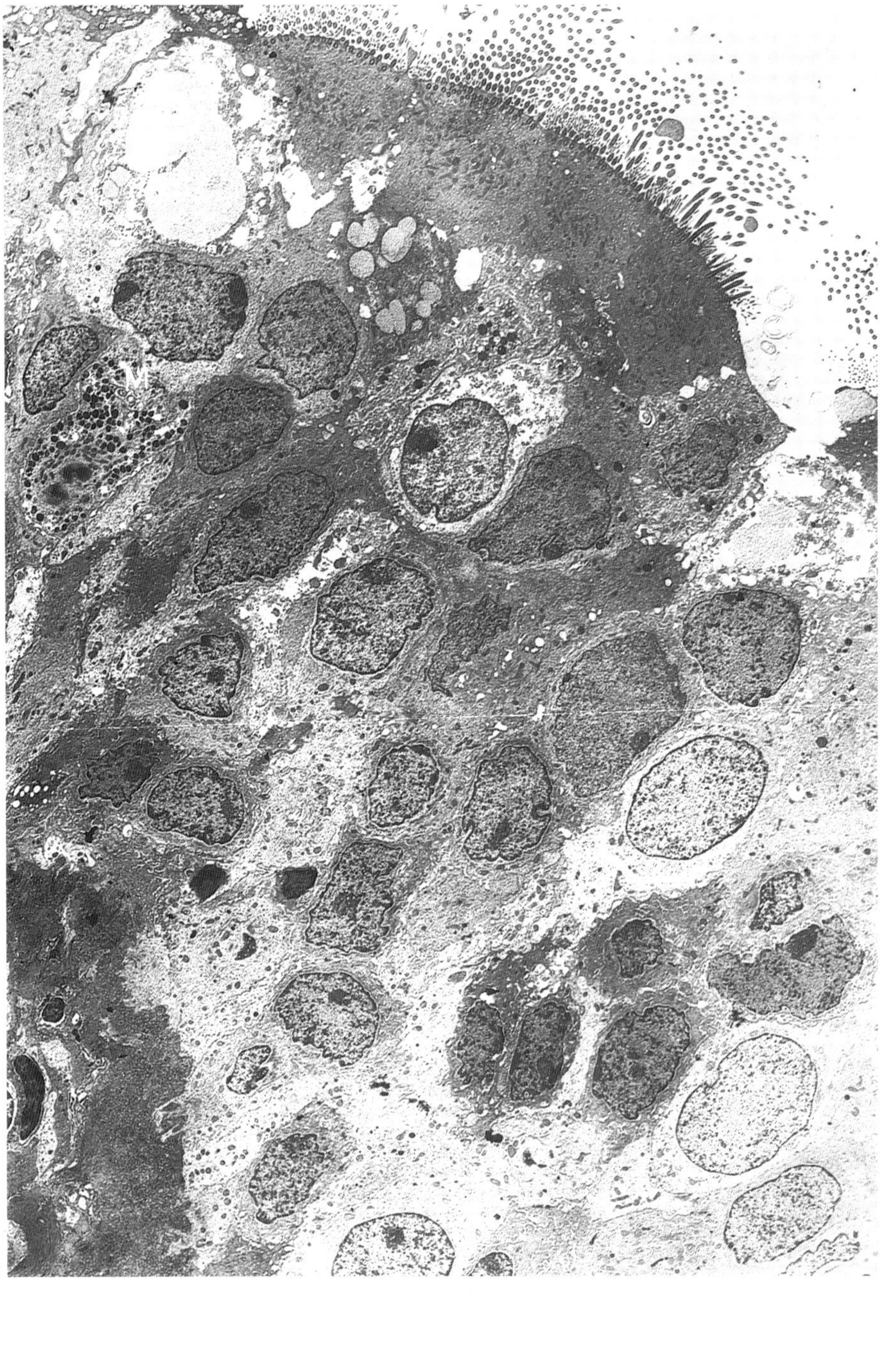

a:

Fig. 27: Intraepithelial lymphocyte.
The normal bronchial mucosa contains irregularly distributed individual lymphocytes (Ly) in the surface epithelium.

TEM
Magnification: 7,500:1

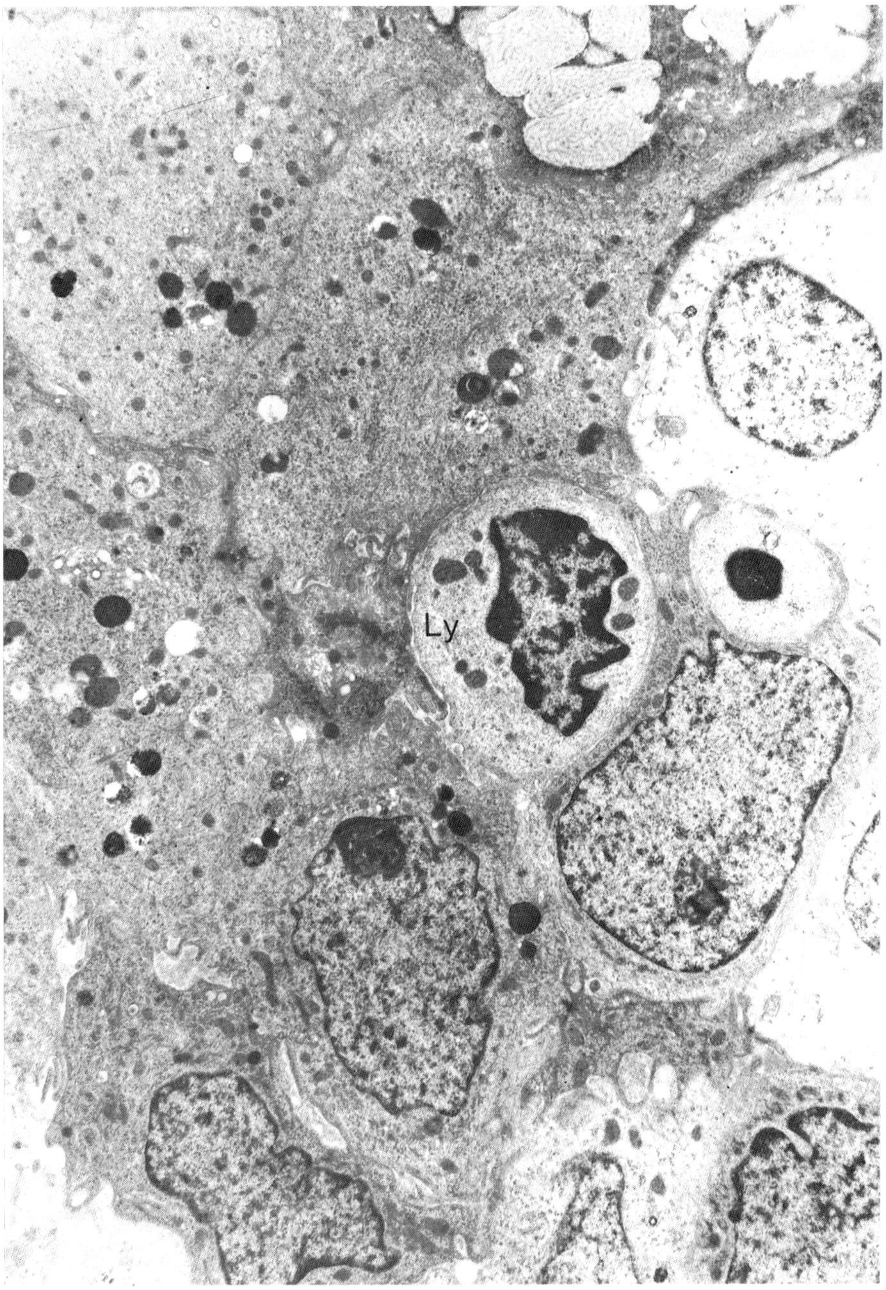

2.7. Structure of the Bronchiolar Mucosa

The bronchiolar epithelium consists of two layers, whereas more peripheral airways have a wall consisting only of one layer. Goblet cells are rare and in the normal terminal bronchioles they are completely absent. Bronchiolar epithelium consists of ciliated cells and Clara cells. Morphologically, the bronchiolar ciliated cells are similar to those of the bronchial epithelium, although they are somewhat shorter. Towards the end of the terminal bronchiole the relative number of ciliated cells decreases progressively.

Fig. 28: Branching respiratory bronchioles cut tangentially.
The numerous dome-shaped projections are the secretory caps of the Clara cells.

SEM
Magnification: 620:1

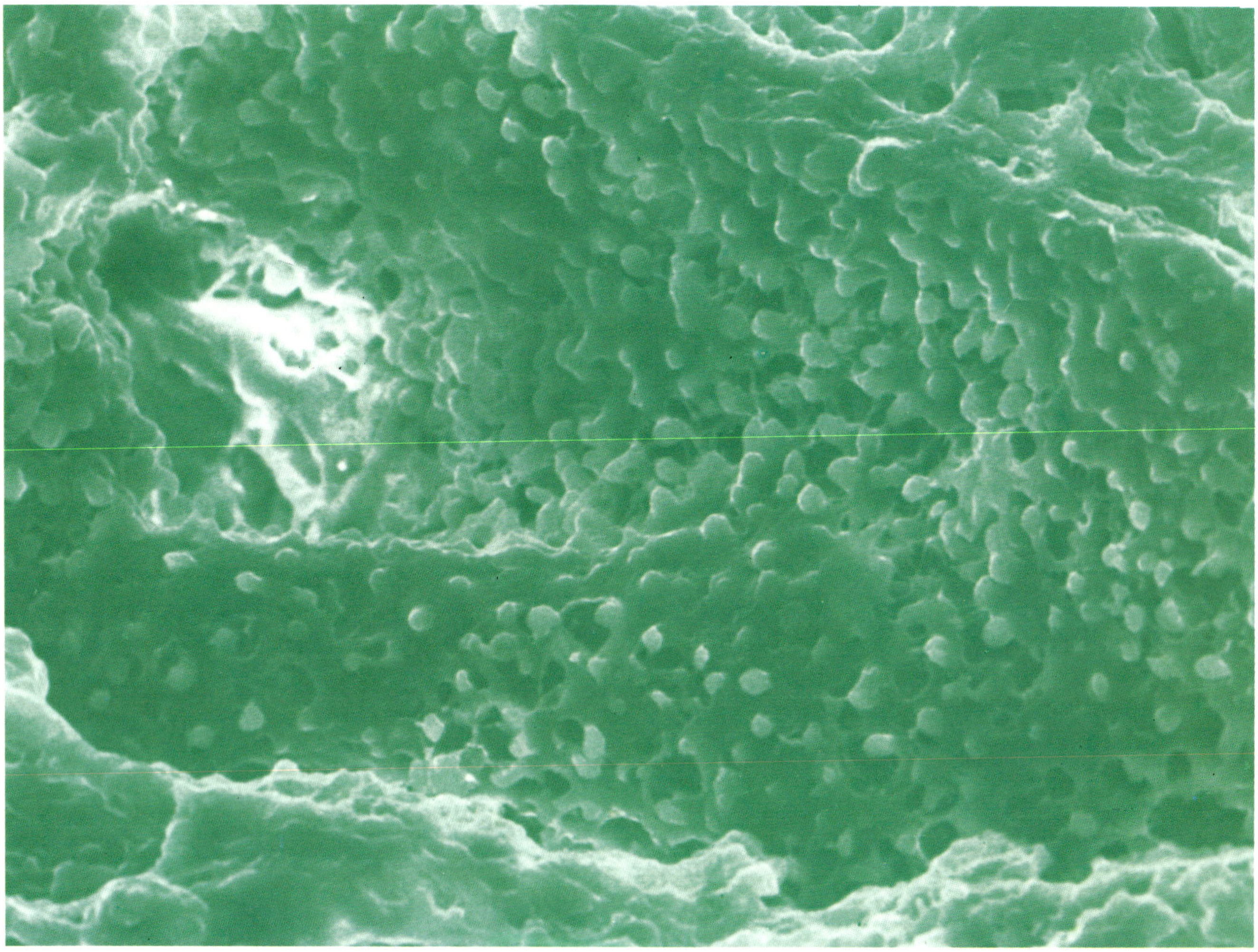

2.7.1. Clara Cells

In a detailed description of the bronchiolar epithelium published in 1937, Clara described non-ciliated cells whose apical caps protruded into the airway lumen. In the proximal bronchioles, Clara cells are only rarely seen, and as the ciliated cells decrease in number in the terminal bronchioles, their number increases and they constitute the majority of the epithelial cells distal to the terminal bronchiole where ciliated cells are absent. Towards the basal zone of the cell, the cytoplasm contains numerous elongated mitochondria, some rough and

Fig. 29: Secretory caps of Clara cells of the bronchiolar epithelium seen after removing the secretory layer. Note uniform, dome-shaped, apical cell projections capable of separating from the cell surface.

SEM
Magnification: 1,320:1

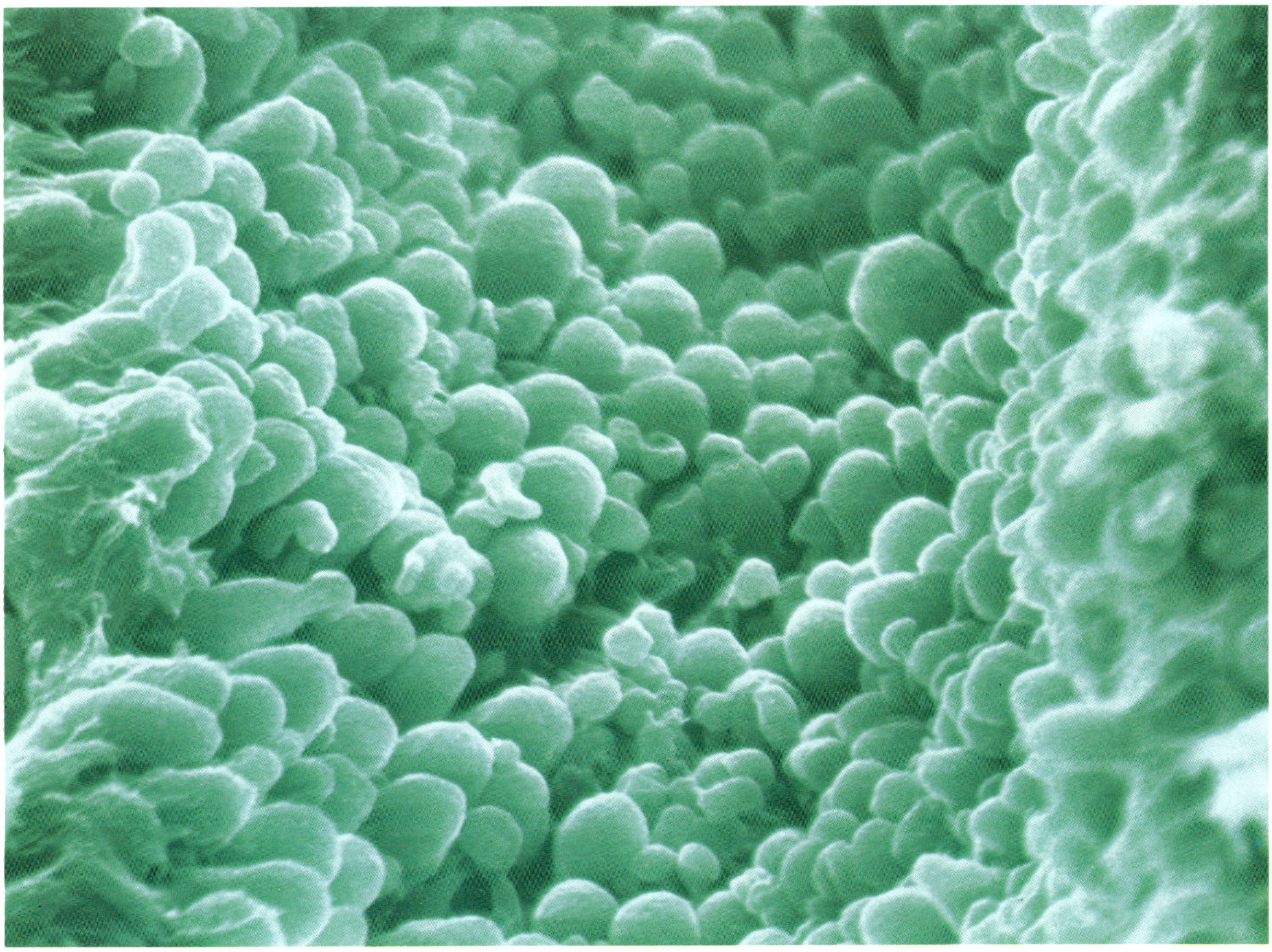

smooth walled endoplasmic reticulum, and free ribosomes. The central zone of the cell contains an elongated nucleus with slender indentations. A Golgi apparatus is almost always seen to one side of the nucleus. The apical zones of the Clara cells bulge into the bronchiolar lumen and are characterized by numerous ductules of smooth endoplasmic reticulum adjacent to which are many mitochondria and lysosomes.

Histochemical investigations of the enzymes in Clara cells have shown a high level of oxydative and, hence, metabolic activity which exceeds that of ciliated or alveolar lining cells. The extent to which Clara cells bulge into the bronchiolar lumen depends upon their maturity. Below the apical cell membrane are found numerous lysosomes and mitochondria. These mitochondria are very dense, relatively small and contain short cristae. With increasing protrusion of the cell apex into the bronchiolar lumen, tubular transformation of the cytoplasm in the apical zone occurs. These tubular structures consist of fine granular material. Beneath the apical cytoplasmic

Fig. 30: Bronchiolar epithelium.
Initial stage of separation of the secretory caps from the Clara cells (arrows). At the junction between the secretory cap and the rest of the cytoplasm, there is an accumulation of mitochondria and lysosomes. The perinuclear zone shows endoplasmic reticulum and the Golgi apparatus.

TEM
Magnification: 10,000:1

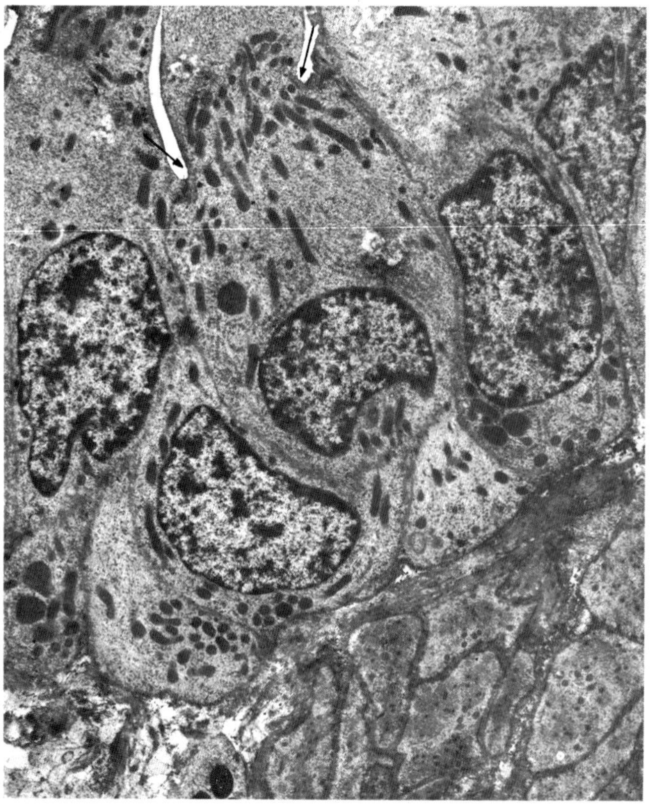

Fig. 31: Cross section of Clara cell secretory cap.
Within the dome-shaped secretory cap there is a uniform tubular cytoplasmic structure. Beneath the cell membrane lysosomes are concentrated, some of which have started to dissolve in the cytoplasm and release their enzymes. The released enzymes probably account for the dissolution of the secretory cap.

TEM
Magnification: 18,000:1

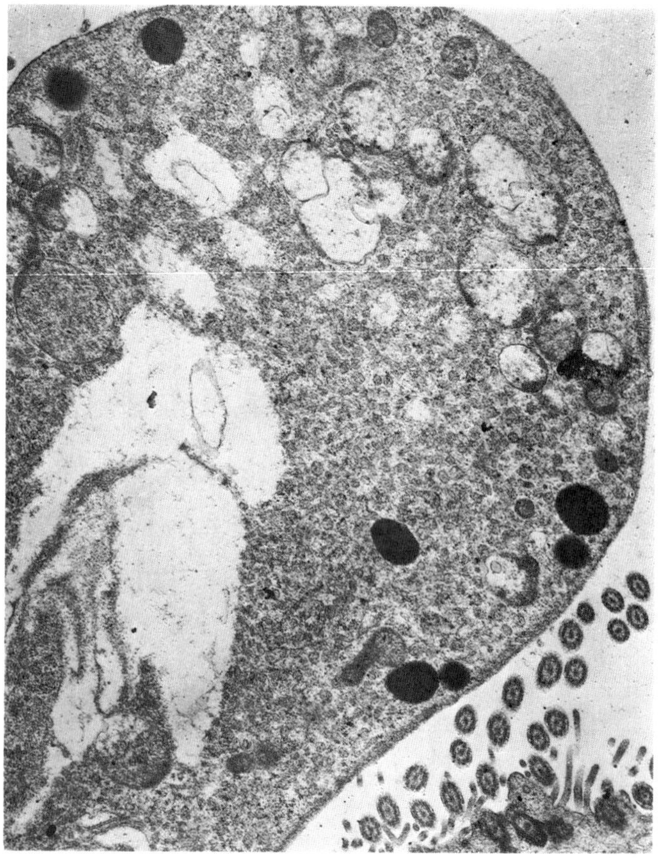

cap, which protrudes deeply into the bronchiolar lumen, the cytoplasm is dense. Beneath the secretory cap which separates zipper-like from the apex of the cell, the new cell membrane forms. The cytoplasmic structure of the now separated apical portion of the cell becomes increasingly indistinct and cloudy, apparently as a result of water absorption, while at the same time, the tubular structures disintegrate. It is likely that the lysosomes which congregate in the apical zone of the cell assist in the disintegration of the apical secretory cap by secreting proteolytic enzymes. It may be that as a result of the enzymatic breakdown of the macromolecular material, there is an increased osmotic gradient favouring uptake of water into the Clara cells, resulting in the observed changes in the apical cap. Eventually, the cap disintegrates totally, its components joining the secretions on the bronchiolar surface. Pathological studies suggest that the serous secretion formed by the Clara cells mixes with the mucous component of the secretions in the more proximal parts of the airway.

Fig. 32: Clara cells showing secretory caps.
Beginning dissolution of the cell membranes (arrows). After separation of the secretory cap and complete dissolution of the cell membrane the contents of the cap become part of the secretory layer on the surface of the bronchiole.

SEM
Magnification: 10,000:1

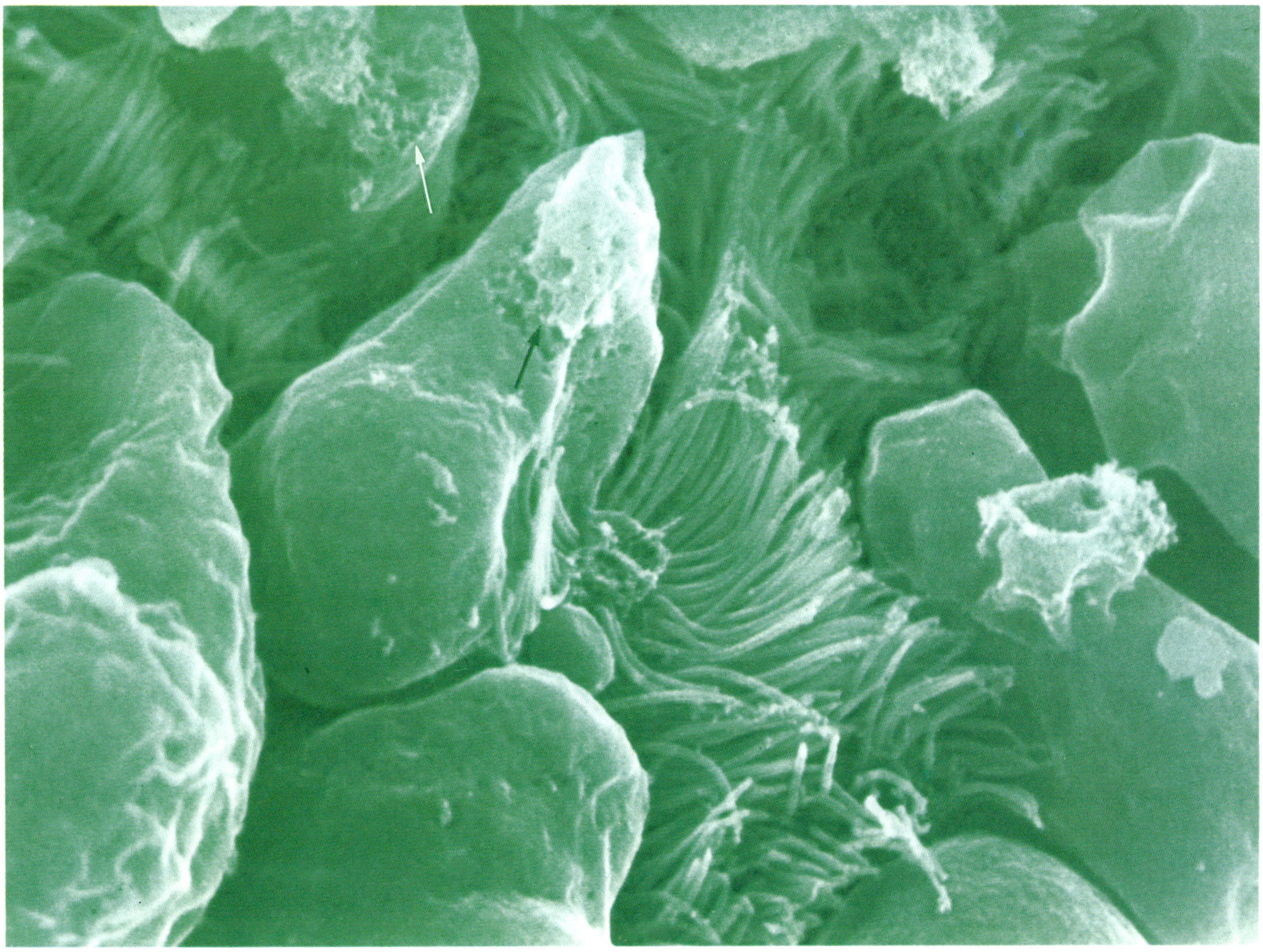

3. Inflammatory Reactions of the Bronchial System

The pathological classification of the inflammatory changes in the bronchial tree is based on the interpretation of the type of inflammatory infiltrate, the composition of the bronchial secretions and inflammatory exudates, as well as the severity of the tissue injury resulting from the inflammatory reaction. The clinical picture of persistent cough and sputum characteristic of respiratory tract hypersecretion is only part of the morphological spectrum of bronchitis. It is, furthermore, important to distinguish between pathophysiological changes in the large and medium-sized bronchi and the changes that occur in more peripheral parts of the airway. Despite the many morphological observations, resulting from innumerable biopsies at various stages of bronchitis in patients with this condition, it is still impossible to develop a rigid classification which allows interpretation of the clinical picture solely from morphological criteria. For this reason, the morphological classification still depends on the clinical course of the illness. On clinical grounds alone, bronchitis is divided into:

1. acute bronchitis
2. chronic bronchitis and
3. bronchiolitis.

3.1. Acute Bronchitis

Acute inflammatory reactions in the bronchial tree tend to involve the entire lower respiratory tract. Commonly, acute bronchitis follows upper respiratory tract infections. However, such episodes may begin as primary tracheitis, bronchitis or bronchiolitis. These acute illnesses occur particularly commonly and severely in infants, young children and the elderly, often with serious sequelae. Infants are probably affected because of their, as yet, poorly developed immune system. In the elderly, the aging immune system, as well as predisposing underlying disease, such as chronic bronchitis or emphysema, may account for the severity of what in young adults might merely be transient and rapidly resolving acute bronchitis. In patients with S-IgA or IgG deficiency, recurrent bronchopulmonary infections are common as a result of immunoglobulin deficiency. Furthermore, recurring episodes of acute tracheobronchitis may result from congenital abnormalities such as primary ciliary dyskinesia or cystic fibrosis or acquired problems such as thermal or chemical injuries, aspiration of refluxed gastric juice and infection. In many cases, there is a combination of various factors which may disturb the defence mechanisms of the bronchial mucosa and/or interfere with mucociliary transport or mucus secretion so

Table 1: Respiratory viruses

Family	Virus	Types	Nucleic Acid
Picornaviridae	Entero		RNA
	Polio	3	
	Coxsackie	30	
	Echo	30	
	Rhino	100	
Reoviridae	Reo	3	RNA
Orthomyxoviridae	Influenza	A B C	RNA
Paramyxoviridae	Parainfluenza	4	RNA
	Mumps	1	
	Measles	1	
	Respiratory Syncytial	1	
Coronaviridae	Corona	1	RNA
Adenoviridae	Adeno	33	DNA

that the integrity of the bronchial mucosa is altered, predisposing to colonization of the airway by inhaled organisms. Inhaled environmental pollutants such as ozone, nitrogen oxides or sulphur dioxide, associated with contemporary urban life, may sometimes predispose to acute respiratory tract illness, particularly in the very young, the elderly and those predisposed by virtue of underlying respiratory tract injury, most commonly due to cigarette smoking.

In the occupational setting, or as a result of accidental exposure from damaged transport vehicles, ammonia, nitrogen oxides, chlorine, etc. may be inhaled in high concentrations resulting in severe and widespread airway epithelial necrosis and serious pulmonary disease or death.

In the airway, the main organisms accounting for bacterial infections include:

- pneumococci
- streptococci
- staphylococci
- haemophilus influenzae
- pseudomonas aeruginosa
- micrococcus catarrhalis and other pyogenic organisms.

The inflammatory reaction is invariably associated with purulent secretions and occasionally when the reactions are very severe, there is associated necrosis.

Viruses account for about 90 % of all acute bronchitic episodes. Table 1 shows the most important viruses.

Viral infections affecting the respiratory tract may be acquired as a result of inhalation of droplet aerosols, but more recent evidence suggests that the majority may be transmitted by direct contact. Furthermore, the respiratory tract may be affected selectively following a viraemia. Frequently, airway viral infections are followed within a few days by secondary bacterial colonization.

The cellular reaction to viruses in the respiratory mucosa consists mainly of accumulations of lymphocytes. There is little associated increase in bronchial secretions. If the inflammatory response is mainly leukocytic, bacterial superinfection is present.

Bronchitis and bronchiolitis caused by viral infections frequently result in proliferation of the epithelium with marked dysplasia.

The prognosis of viral bronchitis and bronchiolitis is usually excellent and complications are almost always the result of secondary bacterial infection. Occasionally, bronchiolitis obliterans occurs, causing a very serious illness, sometimes resulting in death or, if recovery occurs, there may be residual, often severe, chronic life-long impairment of pulmonary function. While viral culture or serological reactions may establish the aetiology of the viral bronchitis, this information is still largely academic, although in recent years, promising developments in the treatment of severe viral respiratory tract infections with systemic or aerosolized antiviral antibiotics offer hope for future successful treatment of these conditions.

In children, viral respiratory tract infections may result in life-threatening illnesses due to bronchiolitis or acute laryngotracheal obstruction.

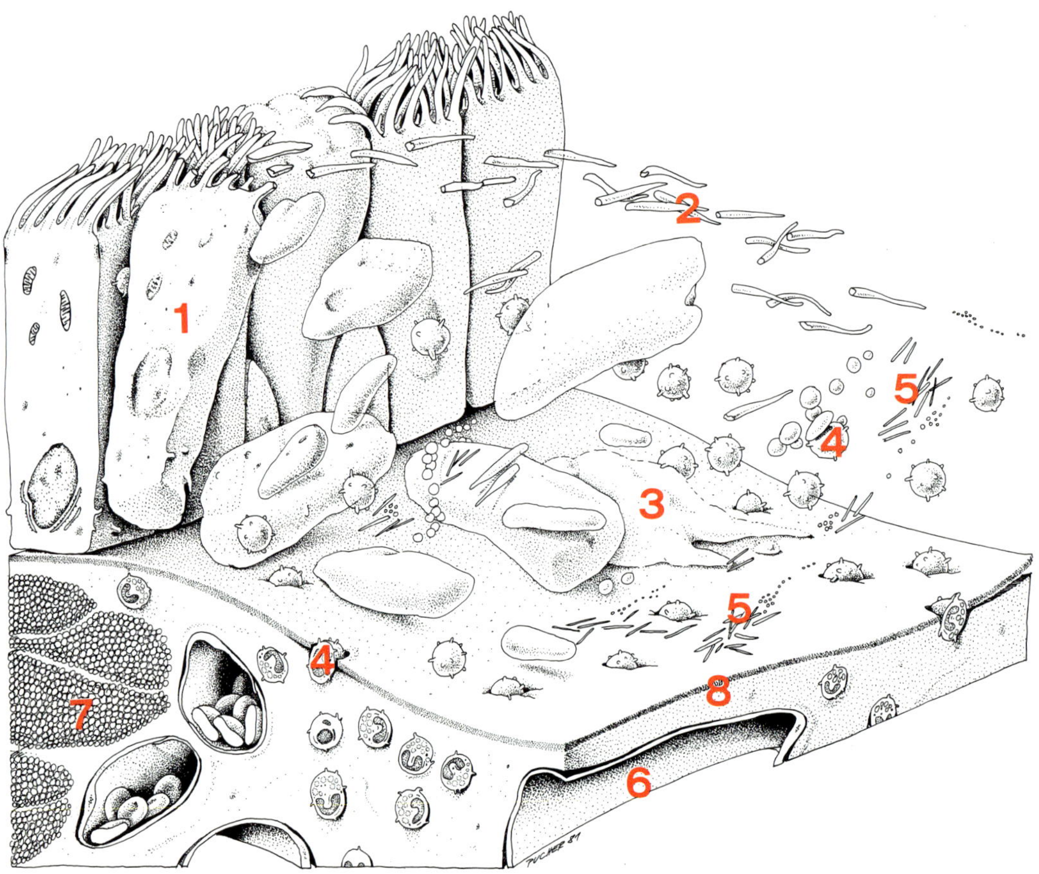

Fig. 33: Three-dimensional diagram of changes in the surface epithelium in acute bronchitis.

1: lucent and partly necrotic ciliated cells
2: ciliary fragments in the bronchial secretion
3: mucus in the gland duct of a peribronchial gland
4: submucosa and basal lamella showing migrating leukocytes
5: bacteria in the bronchial secretions
6: blood vessels of the bronchial wall
7: smooth muscle
8: basal lamella of the surface epithelium

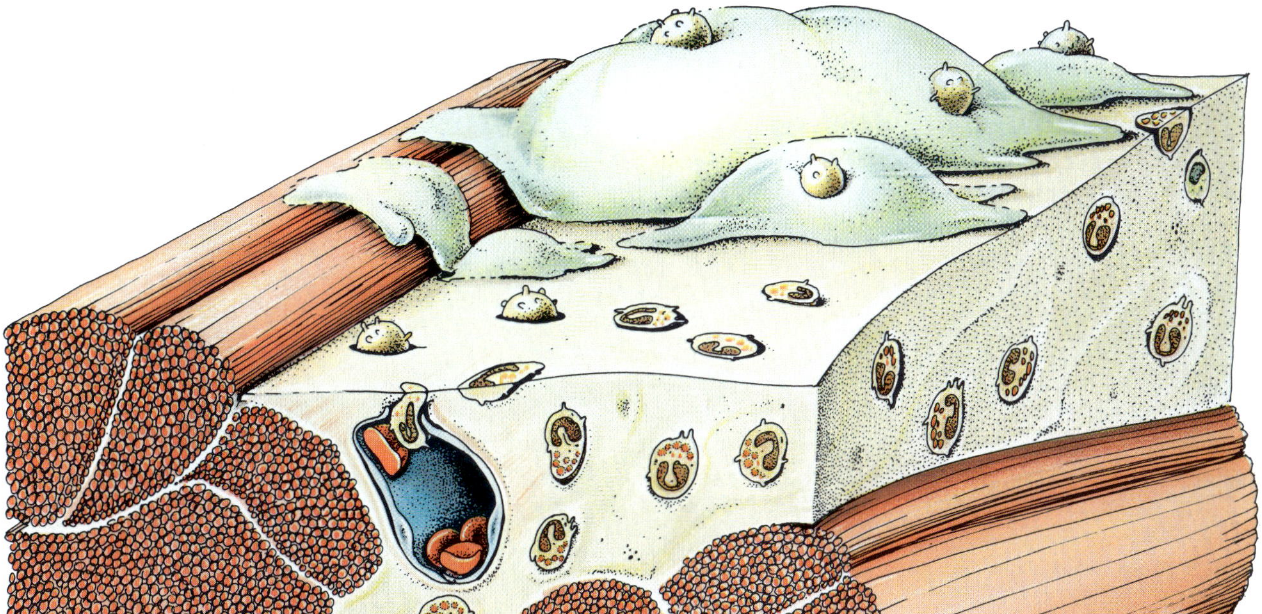

3.1.1. Morphology of Acute Bronchitis

Morphologically, acute bronchitis can be divided into:

1. catarrhal (mucopurulent),
2. fibrinous (pseudomembranous),
3. necrotizing (ulcerative) types.

3.1.1.1. Catarrhal (mucopurulent) bronchitis

In acute catarrhal bronchitis, the bronchial mucosa is hyperaemic and oedematous. The inflammatory reaction may evolve with the production of relatively little tenacious secretion or, alternatively, may run a more productive course characterized by copious seromucous secretions, derived in part from the goblet cells of the surface epithelium and, in part, from the submucosal glands. Additional serous exudate may come from the dilated mucosal capillaries. As a result of this exudation, the surface epithelium is loosened and lifted away from the basal membrane. The exudate is usually rich in leukocytes. Due to overproduction of secretions and exudation as well as bronchospasm, airways obstruction and focal abnormalities of ventilation occur. These changes are fully reversible.

Fig. 35: Acute mucopurulent bronchitis.
Cross section of an obstructed bronchus containing a mucous plug. The mucous plug is densely infiltrated with leukocytes and occasional bronchial epithelial cells.

LM
Stain: Hematoxylin-eosin
Magnification: 850:1

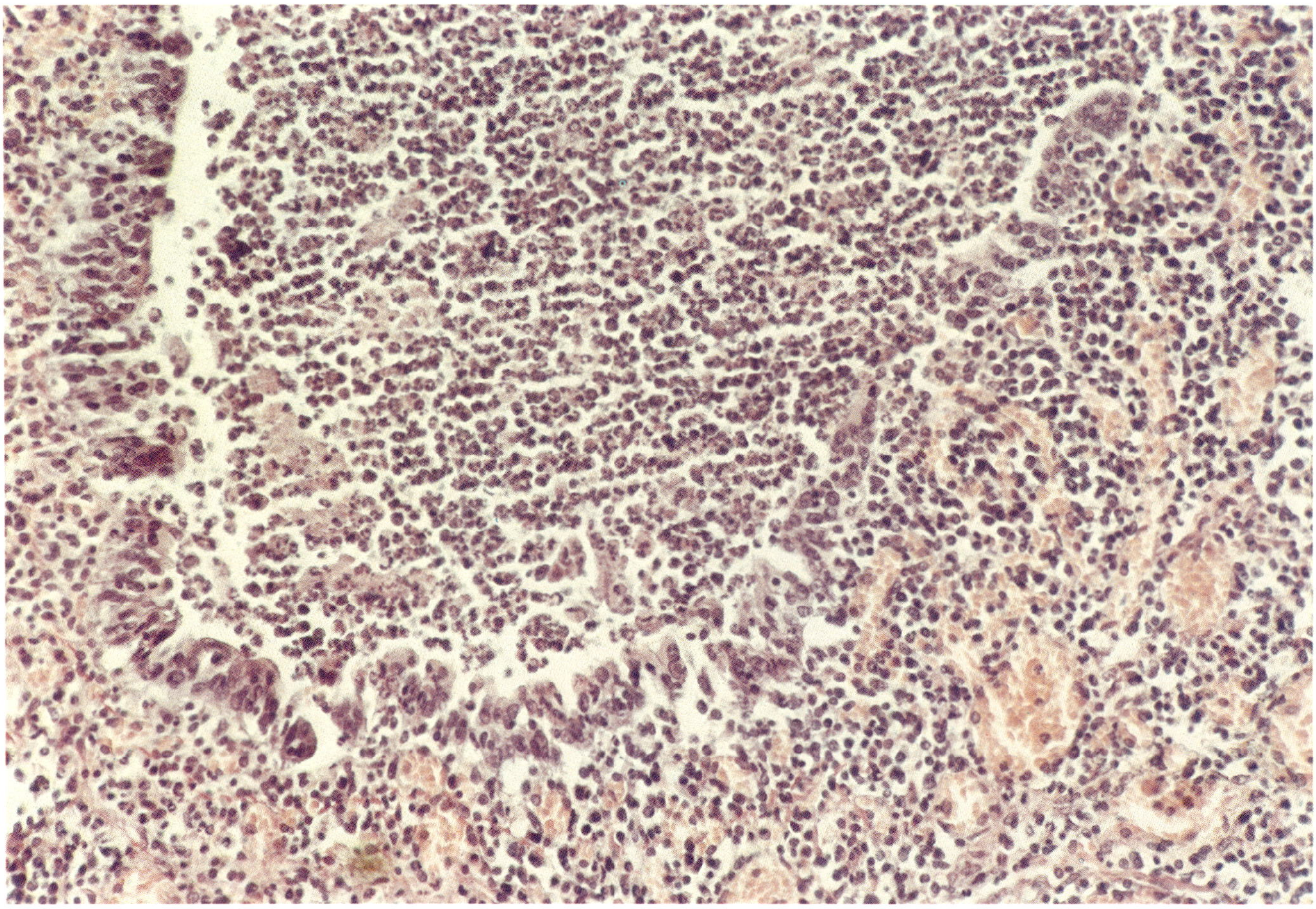

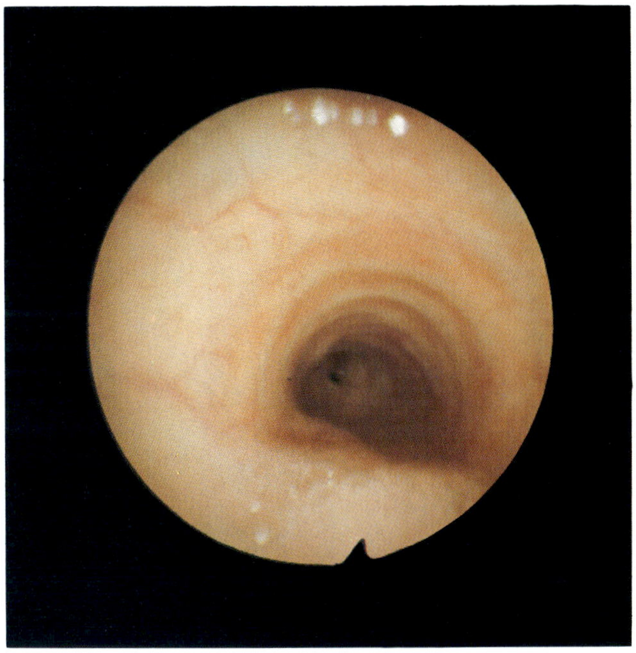

Fig. 36: Acute bronchitis. Vasodilatation showing a reticular appearance.
Acute bronchitis may present as generalized mucosa oedema and hypersecretion or, as depicted here, as dilatation of mucosa vessels and hyperirritability.

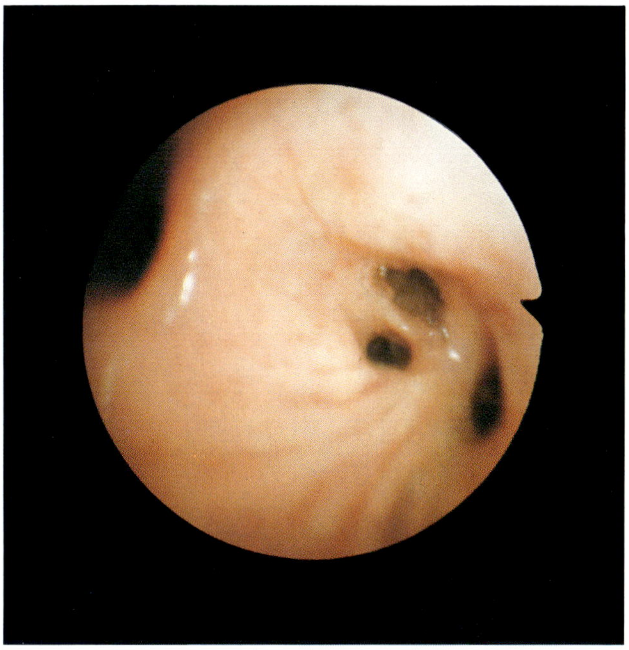

Fig. 37: Acute on chronic bronchitis.
Acute bronchitis superimposed upon early chronic bronchitis shows, in addition to hyperaemia and hypersecretion, a somewhat thickened mucosa and furrowing of the surface (post right upper lobectomy); the stump is seen in the distance).

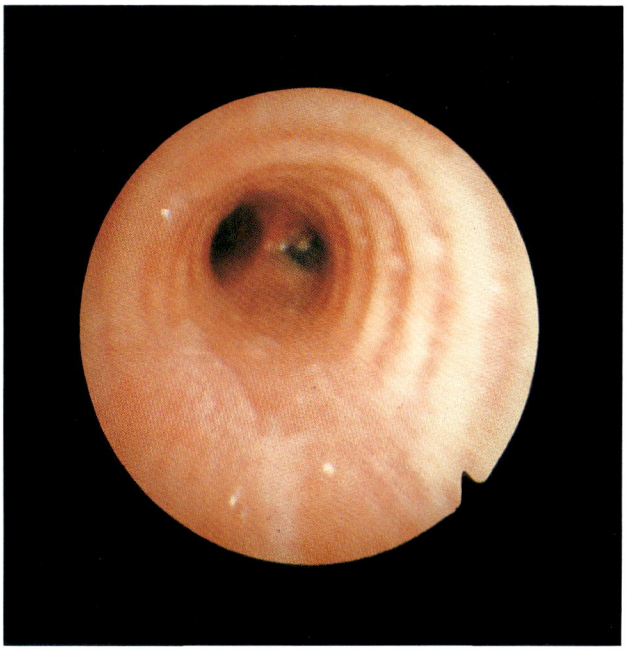

Fig. 38: Acute localized bronchitis.
Mucosal vascular dilatation seen here in the upper lobe bronchus may be an expression of a local acute inflammatory reaction as seen here. If, in addition, there is loss of definition or airway narrowing, carcinoma of the lung should be considered.

Acute fibrino-purulent bronchitis.
Cross section of medium sized bronchus. The bronchial lumen is filled with fibrinous leukocyte-rich mucus.

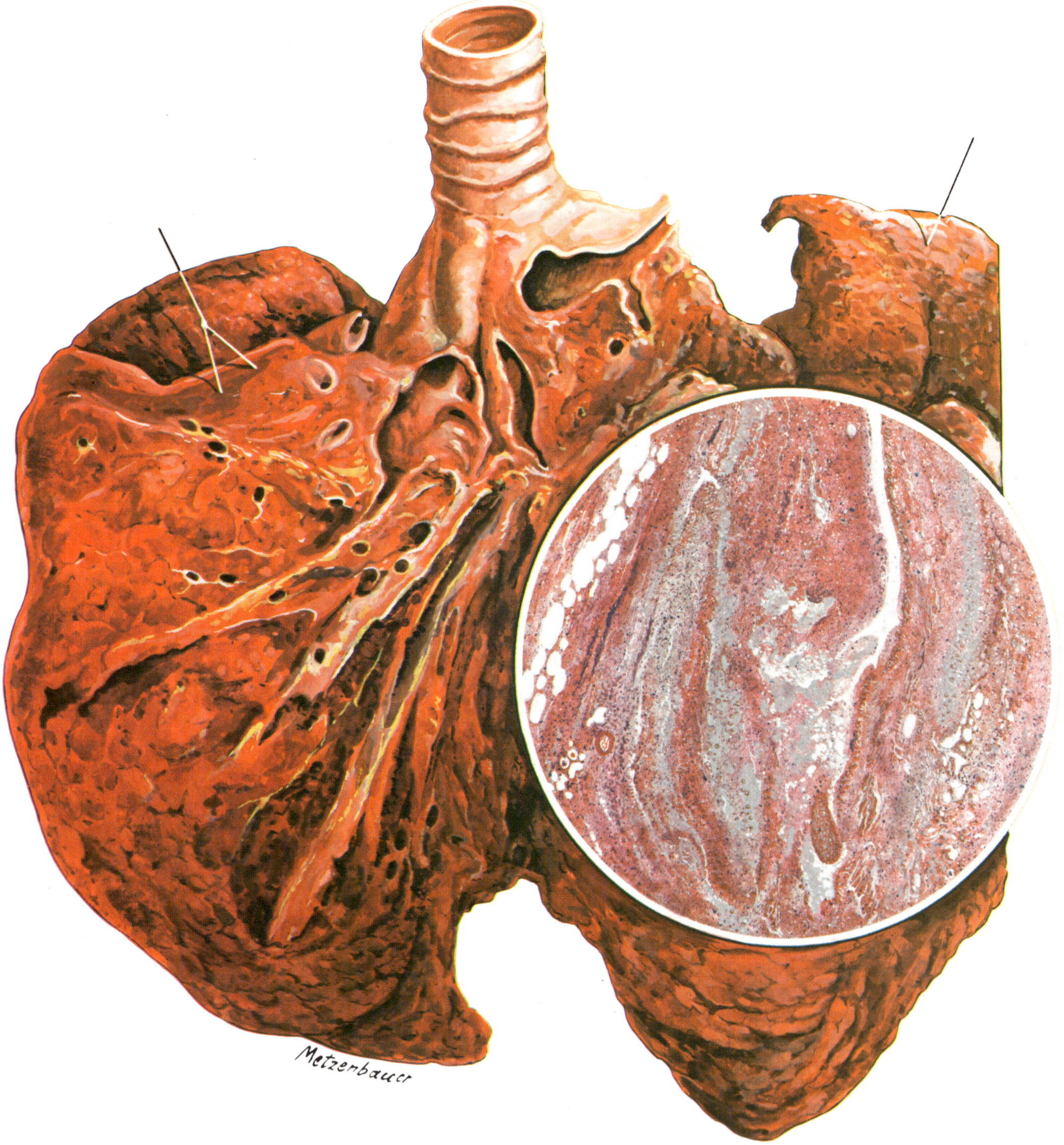

Fig. 39: Acute fibrinous purulent bronchitis. Macroscopic appearance drawn from a pathological specimen. Redness and oedema of the bronchial mucosa extends to peripheral airway branches. The bronchial lumen is filled with purulent secretions. The lung parenchyma shows irregularly distributed patchy areas of poor ventilation.

3.1.1.2. Fibrinous (pseudomembranous) bronchitis

As a result of exudation of fibrinogen onto the mucosal surface, pseudomembranes may develop which may completely obstruct the lumen of small bronchi. These pseudomembranes may be completely cleared as a result of cough. In the now very rare condition of diphtheria, which usually produces severe upper airway obstruction, extensive fibrinous exudate may cause severe and life-threatening obstruction even in peripheral airways.

3.1.1.3. Necrotizing (ulcerative) bronchitis

Necrosis of the bronchial mucosa can result from the inhalation of corrosive gases, aspiration of gastric contents or foreign bodies, endotracheal tubes used for prolonged periods of assisted ventilation and severe bacterial or viral infections. The necrotic mucosa is sloughed off leaving areas of ulceration, following which mucosal regeneration may occur. Within a relatively short period of as little as three to seven days, regeneration of the bronchial epithelium begins, with development of a columnar or squamous epithelium, at first relatively undifferentiated, but this later differentiates into a completely normal bronchial epithelium, consisting of ciliated and goblet cells. If the mucosal injury is severe with ulceration extending through the basement membrane, regeneration of a normal epithelium does not occur, instead, there is a fibroblastic reaction, frequently with extensive scarring.

Fig. 40: Acute necrotizing bronchitis.
Widespread necrosis of the bronchial mucosa with bacterial colonization of the secretions and detritus on the mucosal surface. The submucosa contains a dense leukocytic infiltration.

LM
Magnification: 420:1

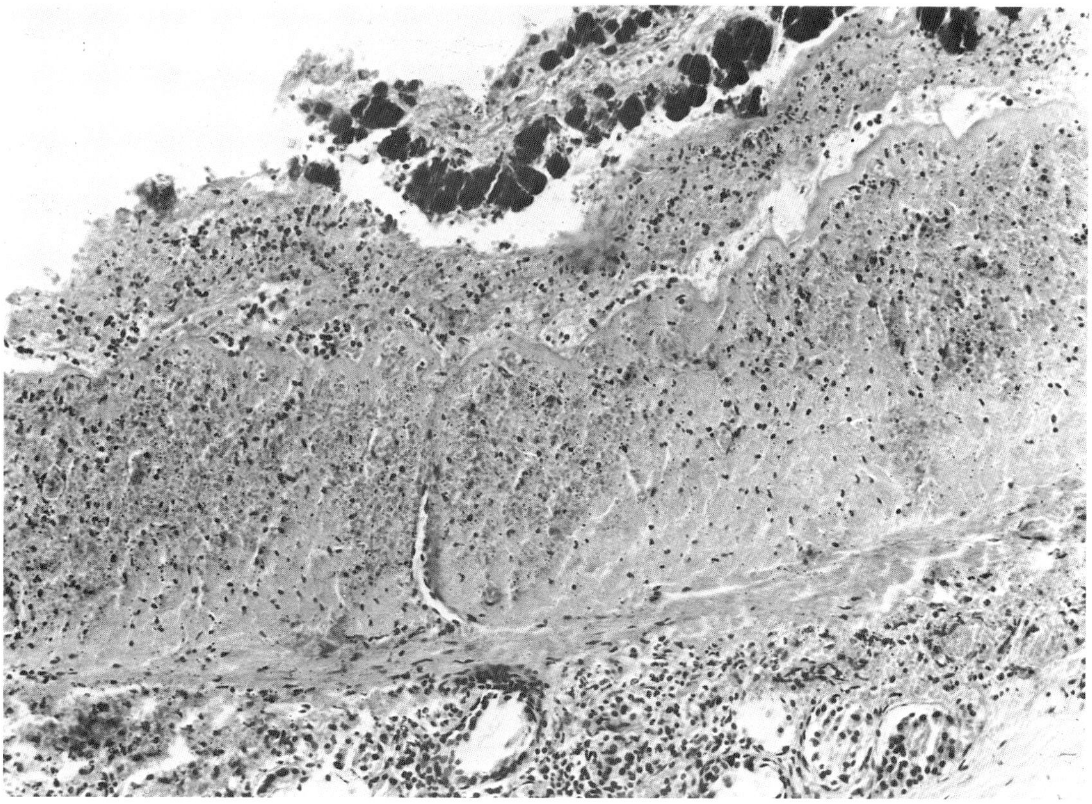

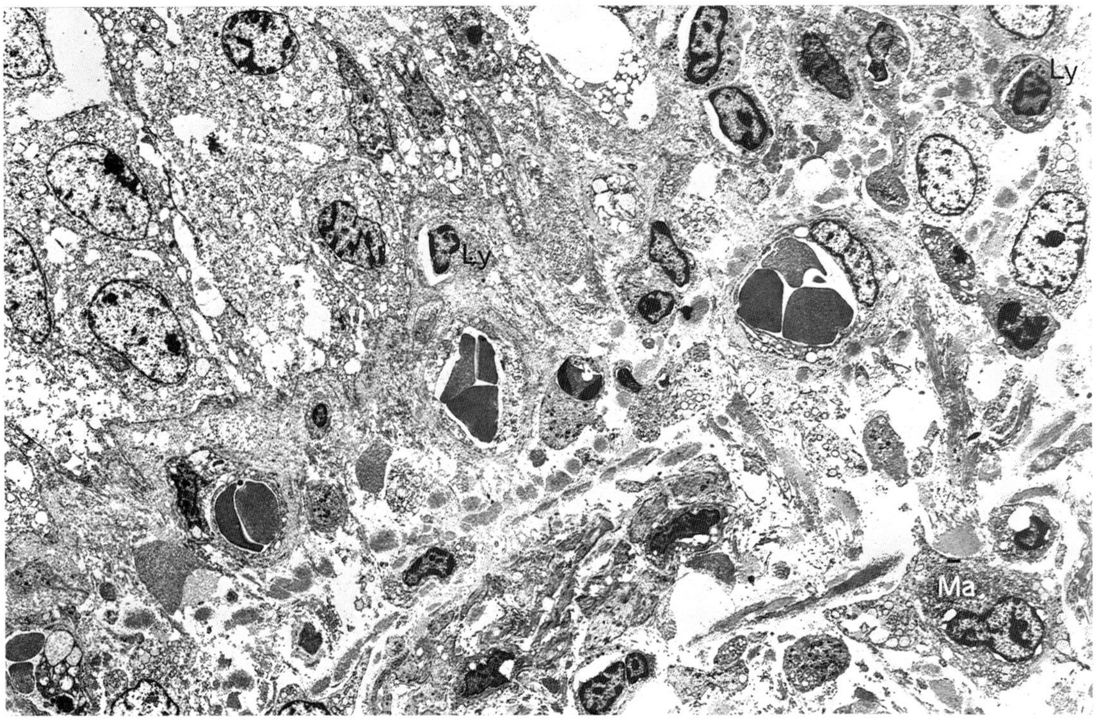

Fig. 41: Necroses of the bronchial epithelium in a fatal case of acute bronchitis and bronchiolitis due to viral infection in a child. Mitochondria show vacuolar degeneration of the epithelial cells. Patchy increased density and focal oedematous dissolution of the cytoplasmic matrix of the bronchial epithelial cells. Widened intercellular spaces. Oedematous swelling of the peribronchial connective tissue and infiltration with lymphocytes (Ly) and macrophages (Ma).

TEM
Magnification: 2,100:1

Fig. 42: Changes in the cilia and microvilli in acute necrotizing bronchitis.
Dissolution of the fine granular and fine filamentary ground substance of the cilia. Cilia break. Fragments of cilia enter the secretory stream. Microvilli show irregular swelling but are still intact.

TEM
Magnification: 16,000:1

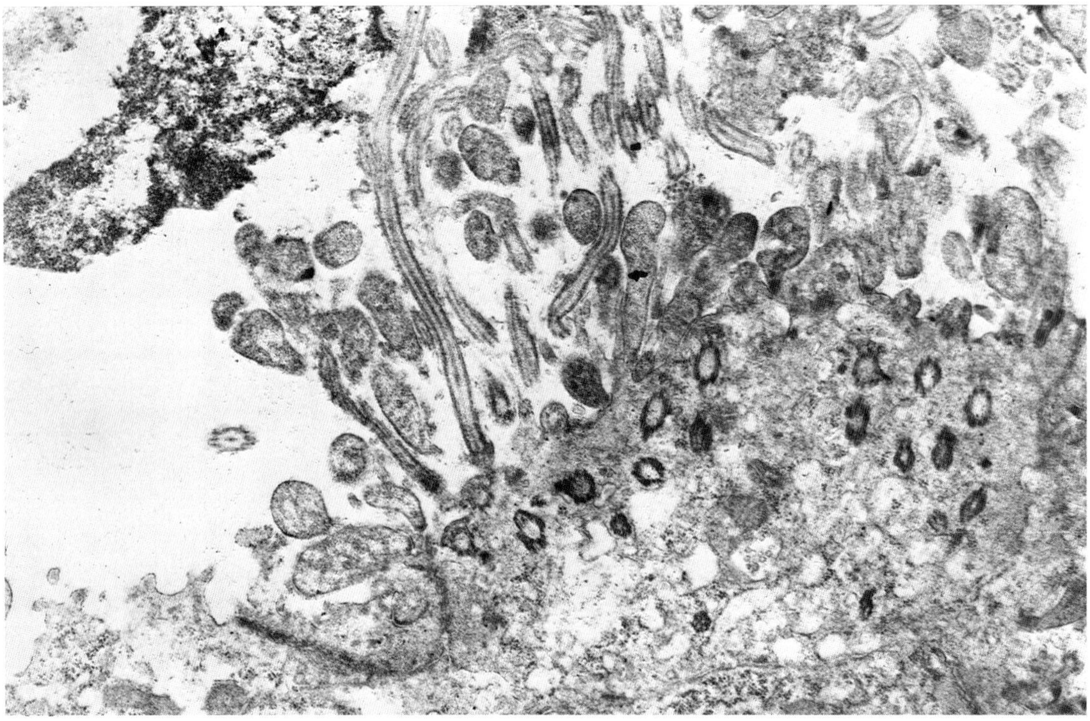

Fig. 43: Extensive loss of cilia on the bronchial surface epithelium in acute necrotizing bronchitis.
The surface epithelium shows a partially intact coarse microvillar structure. Leukocytes (Leu) migrate through the bronchial epithelium.

TEM
Magnification: 16,000:1

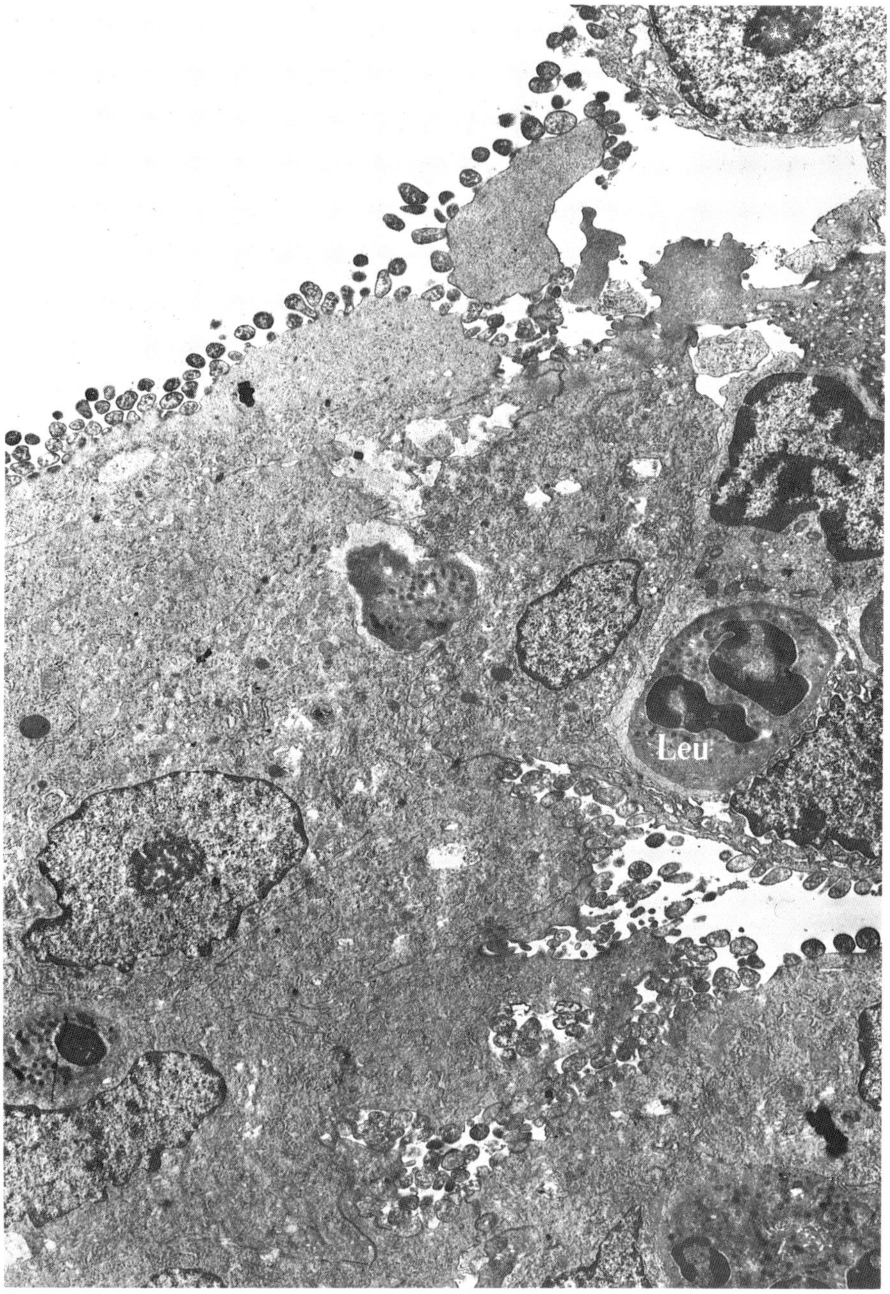

3.2. Bronchiolitis

Severe inflammatory reactions in the terminal segments of the airway frequently lead to major abnormalities of lung function if sufficient peripheral airways are affected. This may be because the gas exchanging portion of the airway is invariably involved and collateral ventilation may be greatly impaired. In this transitional zone from the respiratory bronchioles to the alveolar ducts and alveoli, the narrow airway lumen is readily obstructed as a result of accumulated secretions and inflammatory exudate. Morphologically, the appearance is that of severely impaired ventilation showing areas of focal air trapping adjacent to patchy areas of atelectasis with a lobar distribution. Frequently, bronchiolitis results from distal extension of infection, often moderate, starting in the larger airways. Infants and the elderly are most frequently and severely affected. In children, infection is almost always of viral aetiology with bacterial infection, if it occurs, a late sequela, while in older people bacterial infections occur earlier and tend to be more severe. Morphologically, catarrhal, intramural, obliterative and peribronchiolitis can be distinguished.

Fig. 44: Bronchiolitis.
Inflammatory cells appear on the epithelial surface after migrating through the mucosa. The secretory caps of the Clara cells can be clearly distinguished.

SEM
Magnification: 2,000:1

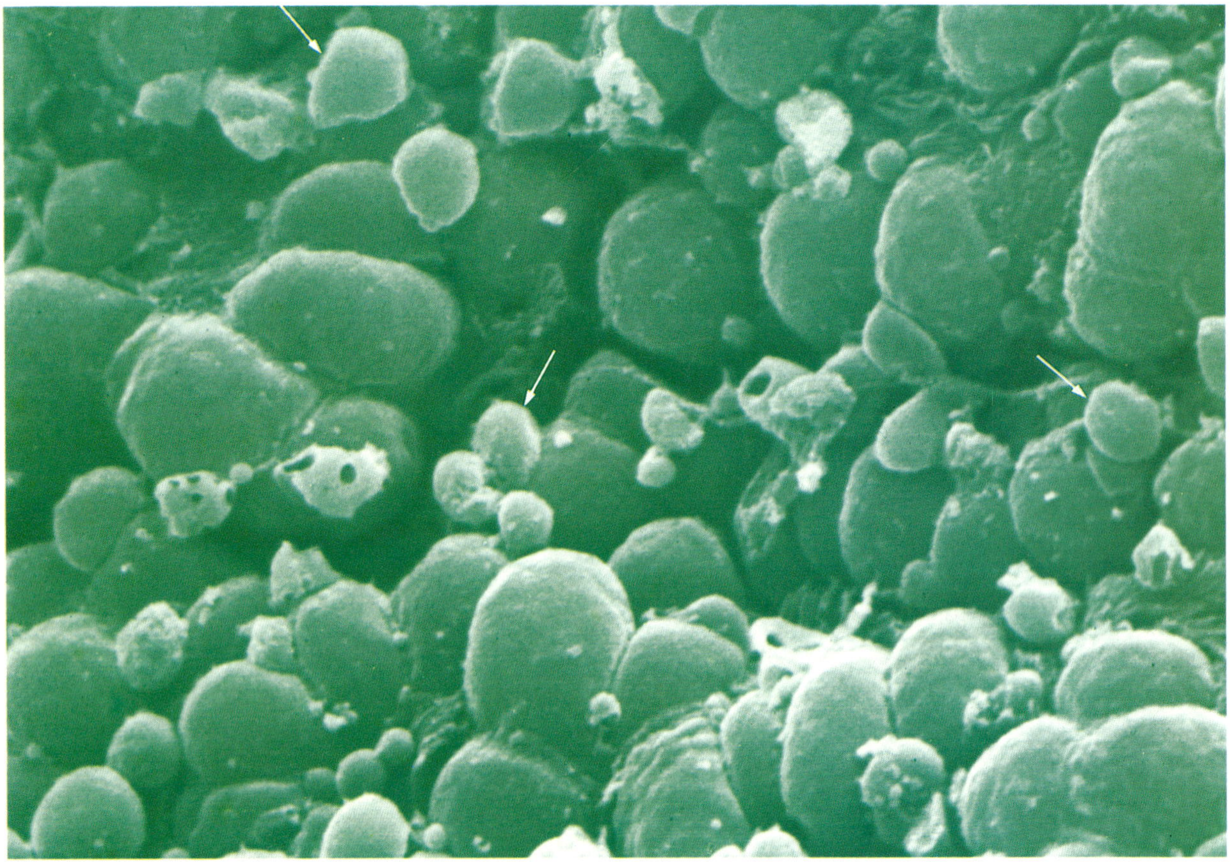

3.2.1. Catarrhal Purulent Bronchiolitis

This condition is characterized by the presence of extremely tenacious secretions consisting of leukocyte-rich exudates, which may completely obstruct the bronchiolar lumen.

3.2.2. Intramural Bronchiolitis

Intramural bronchiolitis is characterized by inflammatory exudates consisting of lymphocytes, plasma cells and monocytes. Frequently, lymphoid follicles develop which narrow the airway lumen. In some cases, histiocytic and reticulocytic infiltrates may be seen which may lead to destruction of the airway smooth muscle and result in scarring. As a result of the destruction of important components of the airway wall, marked impairment of function occurs. Morphologically, it is possible to distinguish between simple (infiltrative), proliferative (epithelial changes) and ulcerative changes in the airway wall (ulcers with tissue destruction and bronchomalacia).

Fig. 45: Acute mucopurulent bronchiolitis.
Complete necrosis of the bronchial epithelium. The lumen is filled with purulent secretions stuffed with polymorpho-nuclear leukocytes and occasional necrotic bronchial epithelial cells.

LM
Semi-thin section
Stain: Basic fuchsin and methylene blue
Magnification: 850:1

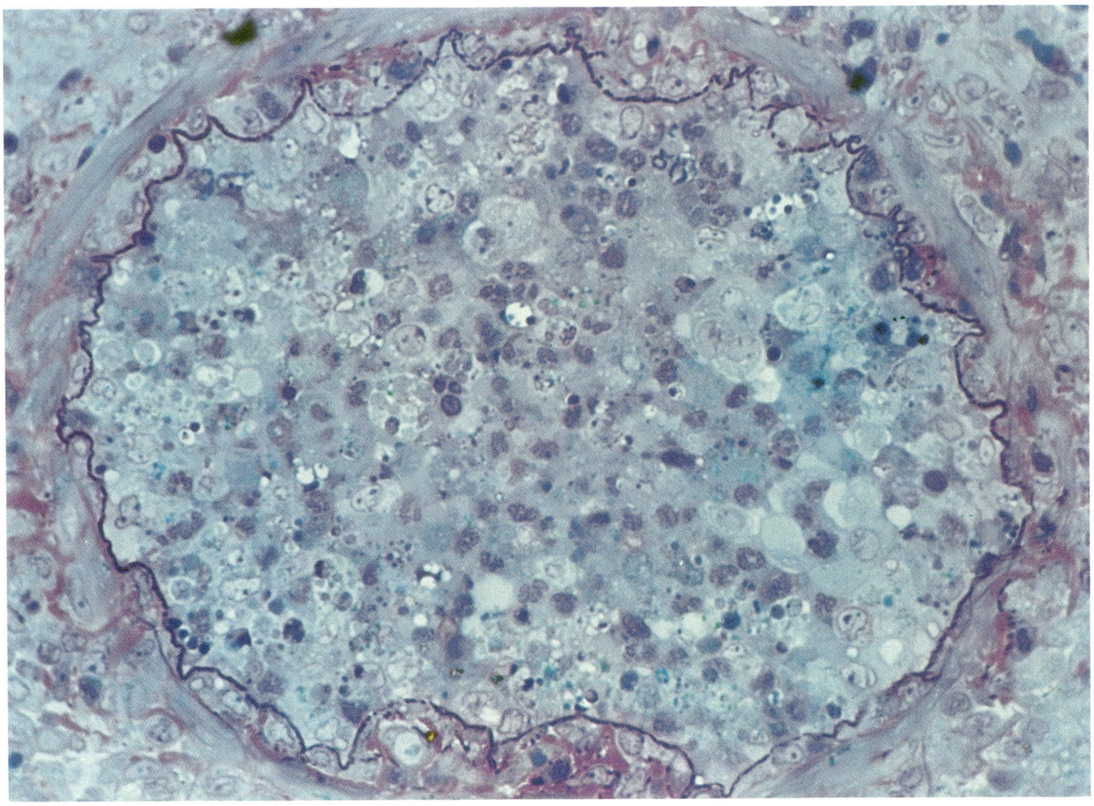

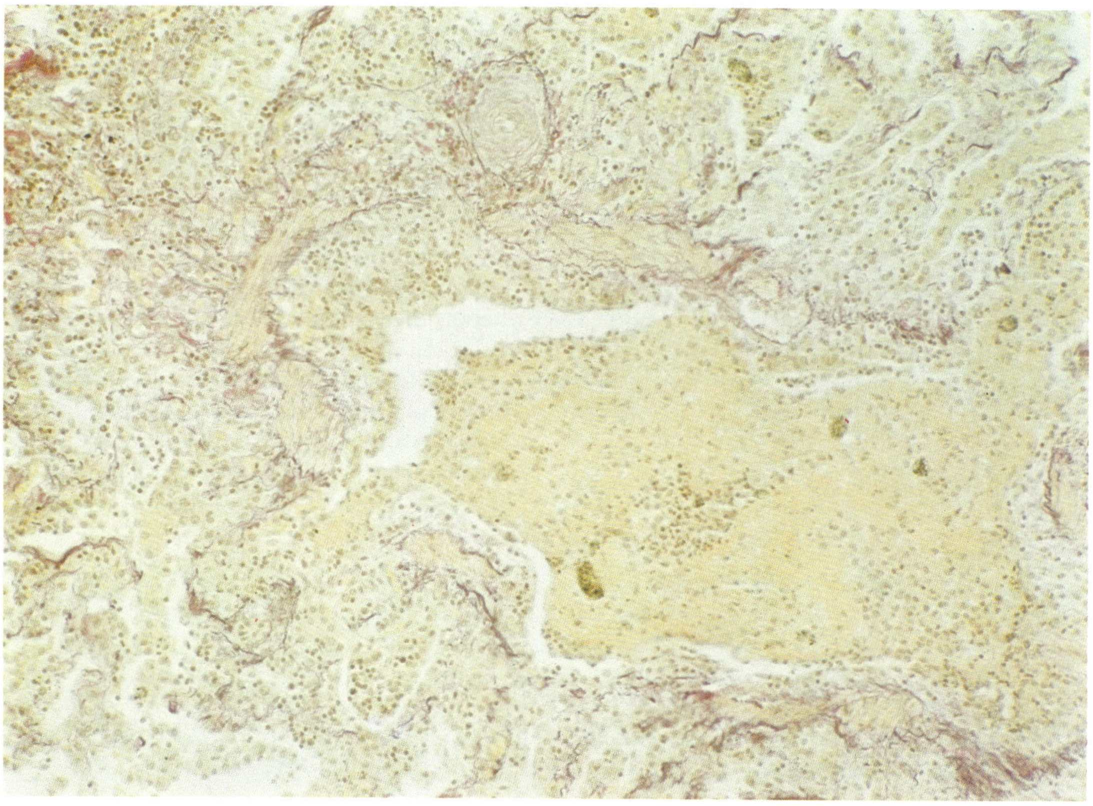

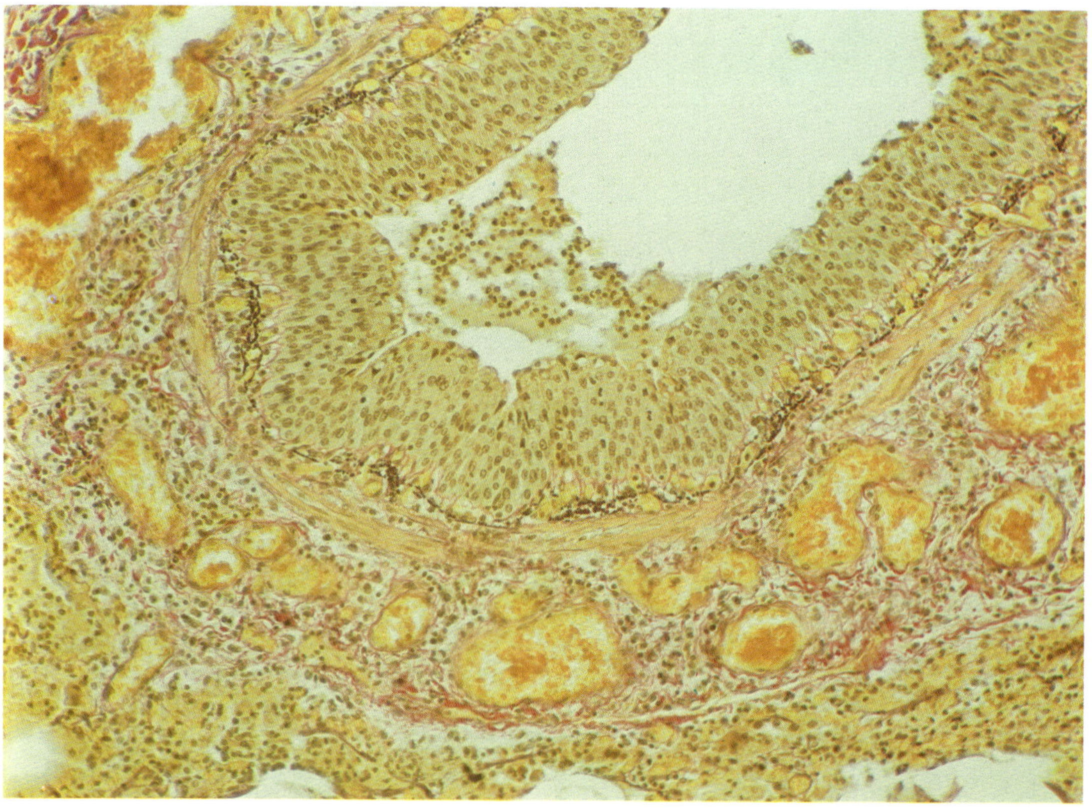

← **Fig. 46:** Acute bronchitis and bronchiolitis due to viral infection. The bronchial lumen is almost completely occluded by a mucous plug. During virus infections, bronchial epithelial cells may transform into giant cells.

LM
Stain: van Gieson
Magnification: 420:1

← **Fig. 47:** Acute bronchitis and bronchiolitis resulting from a virus infection with marked reactive proliferation of the bronchial epithelium. The normal pseudostratified epithelial structure has been lost. Predominantly lymphocytic infiltration of the submucosa as well as extensive hyperaemia of the bronchial wall and vasodilatation in the submucosa.

LM
Stain: van Gieson
Magnification: 420:1

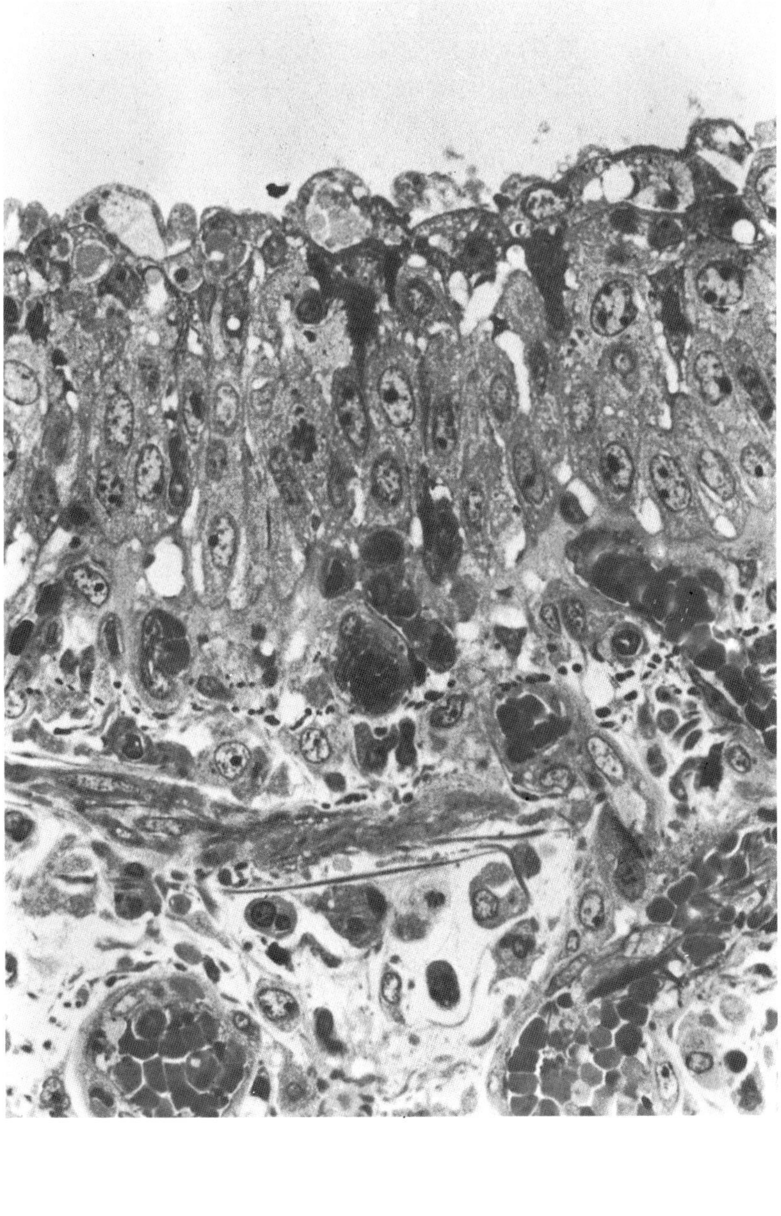

Fig. 48: Acute viral bronchitis.
Reactive proliferation of the bronchial epithelium in acute viral bronchitis. Dysplastic changes may be seen in the epithelium. Increased mitotic figures are seen. The differentiation into ciliated and goblet cells has been lost.

LM
Semi-thin section
Magnification: 1,200:1

3.2.3. Bronchiolitis Obliterans

With the onset of bronchiolitis obliterans, the inflammatory reaction is associated with necrotizing and ulcerative changes. As a result of proliferation of connective tissue components in the submucosa and organization of the inflammatory exudate, granulation tissue develops. Consequently, marked narrowing or even complete obstruction of the airway lumen results. In severe cases, the airway may be so severely affected that the patient may die after only a few days because of acute respiratory failure, or alternatively after a somewhat longer period, if the course is subacute. If the patients survive the acute phase, they may be left with residual severe pulmonary dysfunction due to widespread bronchostenosis often associated with bullous emphysema and bronchiectasis.

If severe bronchiolitis develops in the first few years of life, the terminal airways may fail to develop properly and alveolar ventilation may be severely impaired due to widespread bronchiolar stenosis. These changes may be lobar or affect the whole of one lung, a condition known as the Swyer-James-McLeod or unilateral hyperlucent lung syndrome. This condition occurs almost exclusively in children whose clinical course is characterized, in severe cases, by severe dyspnea and cyanosis even at rest. Even though corticosteroid therapy is contraindicated in virus infections, in cases of bronchiolitis obliterans, short term, high dose steroid therapy is often given usually with equivocal results.

Fig. 49: Bronchiolitis obliterans.
The epithelium is, for the most part, lifted away from the bronchial wall as a result of marked oedema between the epithelium and basal membrane. The bronchiolar lumen contains leukocytic exudate and is partially obliterated by granulation tissue.

Stain: van Gieson
Magnification: 850:1

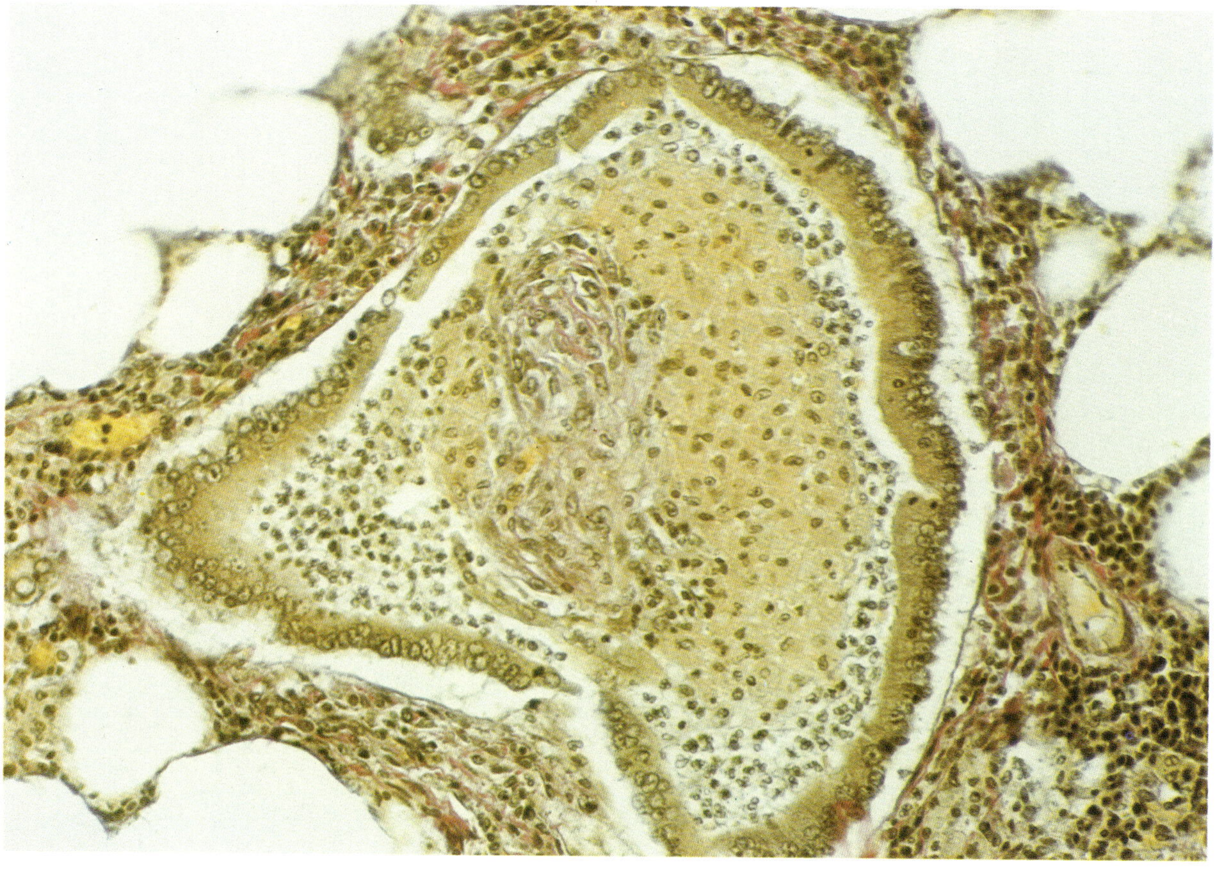

3.2.4. Peribronchiolitis

Peribronchiolitis may be associated with any severe longstanding bronchiolitis. It occurs with considerable frequency in viral infections in children. The inflammatory reaction may spread from the bronchial wall to the peribronchial tissues and thus to the adjacent alveoli. Focal necrotic areas of varying extent and depth with associated areas of reactive proliferation of the bronchial epithelium may be seen. The bronchiolar lumen is greatly narrowed by the inflammatory reaction in the peribronchiolar, intra-acinous and intra-alveolar septa.

The inflammatory infiltrate may extend from the peribronchiolar region to the periphery of the pulmonary lobule. Thus, the alveoli become involved and may become obliterated by inflammatory exudate and desquamated epithelial cells.

Interstitial pulmonary fibrosis may result from the fibroblastic reaction and eventual scarring resulting from the inflammatory reaction and this evolution is frequent following measles and pertussis infections.

Fig. 50: Acute bronchiolitis with extensive peribronchiolitis.
Necroses of the bronchial epithelium. Peribronchial inflammatory cell reaction with infiltration of the peribronchial connective tissue with lymphocytes and macrophages.

LM
Semi-thin section
Stain: Basic fuchsin and methylene blue
Magnification: 750:1

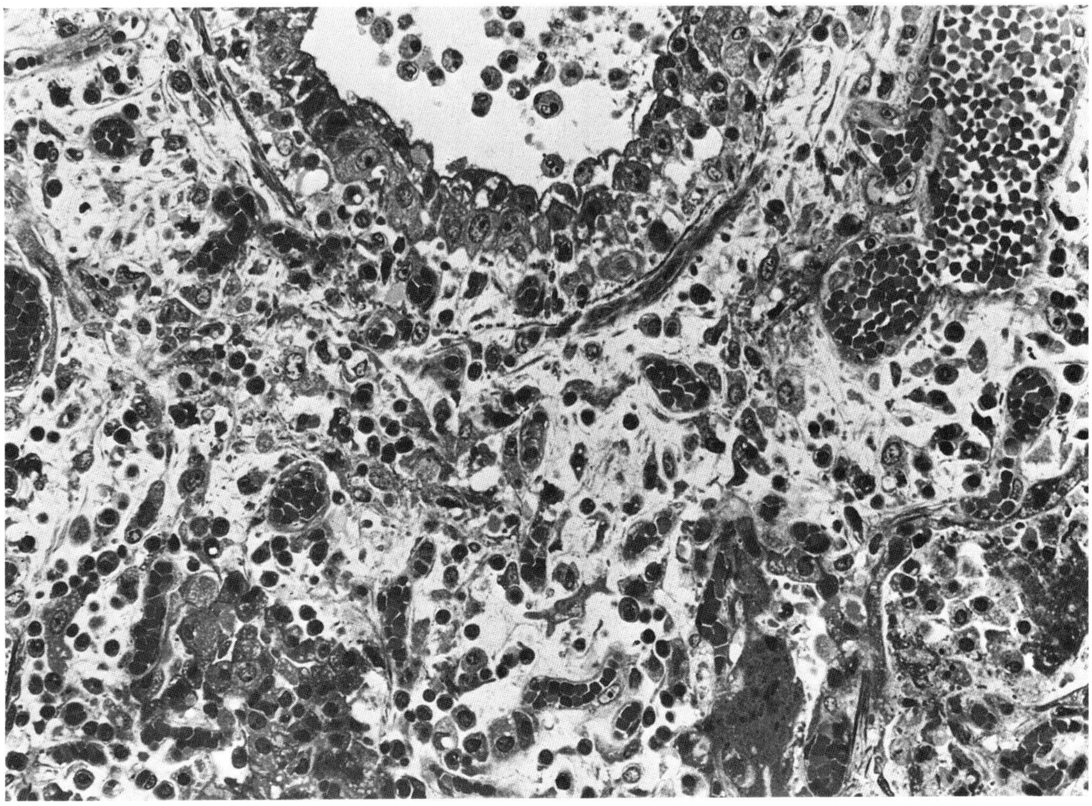

3.3. Chronic Bronchitis

The aetiology of chronic bronchitis remains uncertain. It is generally thought that the condition results from a combination of exogenous agents superimposed upon a genetic predisposition resulting in the characteristic clinical picture. The most important factors contributing to the aetiology and pathogenesis of chronic bronchitis include prolonged heavy tobacco smoking, chronic aspiration of gastric contents, occupational and to a much lesser extent environmental pollutants, recurring infections, allergy, and underlying congenital or acquired disease with associated bronchiectasis. Impaired lung defences resulting from such conditions as primary ciliary dyskinesia, cystic fibrosis, impaired humoral or cellular immunity and inhaled foreign bodies may also play a role. Poor socio-economic status characterized by malnutrition and inadequate attention to minor respiratory tract infections and diseased teeth and gums, and impaired upper airway defences resulting from excess alcohol intake, sedation or unconsciousness from any cause as well as chronic sinusitis, may also contribute.

In recent years, the morphological evaluation of chronic bronchitis has been greatly aided by bronchoscopy and transbronchial biopsy. Repeated fiberoptic bronchoscopies and sequential biopsies make it possible to evaluate the pathological features in relation to the severity of the clinical picture.

From the morphological appearance, various types of chronic bronchitis may be classified according to relatively typical morphological criteria. Presumably these merely represent various stages in the course of bronchitis rather than separate diseases.

The following types can be distinguished:

1. catarrhal chronic bronchitis
2. chronic intramural bronchitis
3. hypertrophic bronchitis
4. chronic-destructive bronchitis
5. chronic peribronchitis.

3.3.1. Catarrhal Chronic Bronchitis

This type of chronic bronchitis is characterized clinically and morphologically by changes in mucus producing elements and in the mucus itself. There is an increase in mucus volume and changes in mucus viscosity.

Morphologically, there is an increase in goblet cells of the bronchial epithelium and even more marked changes in the peribronchial glands. The serous components of the glandular acini disappear leaving only the mucus forming elements. In addition, goblet cells are found with increasing frequency in the mucous gland ducts. Both the mucous gland acini and excretory ducts are dilated and filled with stringy tenacious mucus. With the sudden overproduction of secretion, epithelial cells may die and cytoplasmic fragments may be found in the mucous plugs. Mucosal inflammatory cell infiltrates may be minimal or absent. It is not certain whether the increase in the number of goblet cells in the surface epithelium and the peribronchial gland duct is real or apparent. Morphological findings favour the conclusion that, under these conditions, production of secretion is relatively chaotic rather than the normal sequential and synchronous process. Thus, it is difficult to identify the various stages of the secretory cycle seen under normal circumstances. Virtually all of the goblet cells are in the same phase of the secretory cycle. Furthermore, there are changes in the composition of the secretions covering the bronchial epithelium. The periciliary fluid may be absent in some areas, while at the same time, the gel layer of the mucus may sink towards the epithelial surface. As a result, cilia may become trapped in the mucus and are thus prevented from maintaining a normal beat frequency and co-ordination. Thus mucociliary transport may be greatly decreased or cease completely, resulting in increasing airway obstruction.

Trachea with mainstem bronchi and lymph nodes

Large circle:
Sectioned bronchial branch showing the picture of catarrhal bronchitis.

Small circle:
Seromucous gland of the bronchial wall showing hypertrophied and dilated gland duct filled with secretion.

A. Schematic diagram of an acinus
a) alveolar duct with alveoli
b) respiratory bronchiole
c) terminal bronchiole

B. Normal alveolar duct

C. Alveolar duct and emphysema showing loss of alveolar walls and remnants of alveolar septae

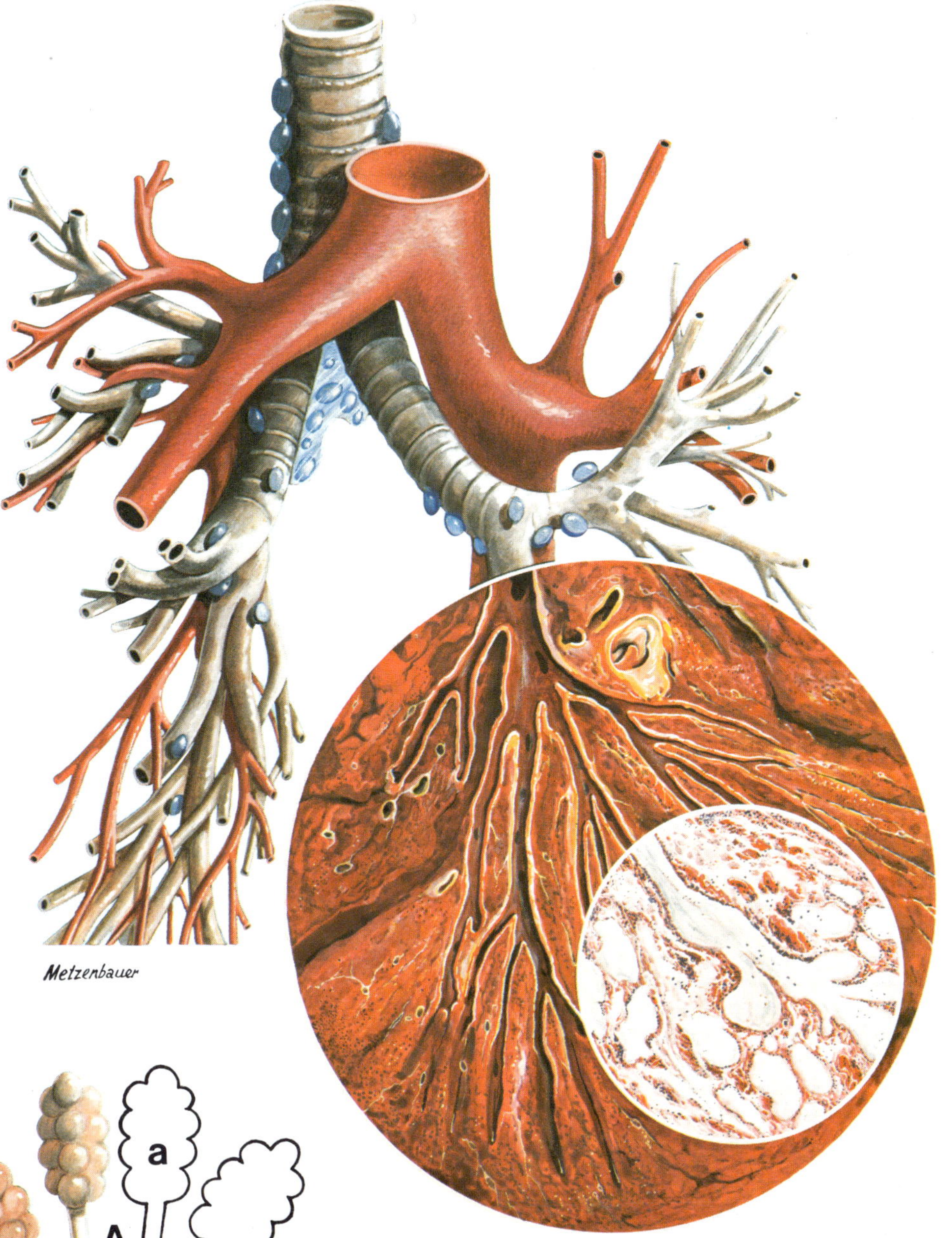

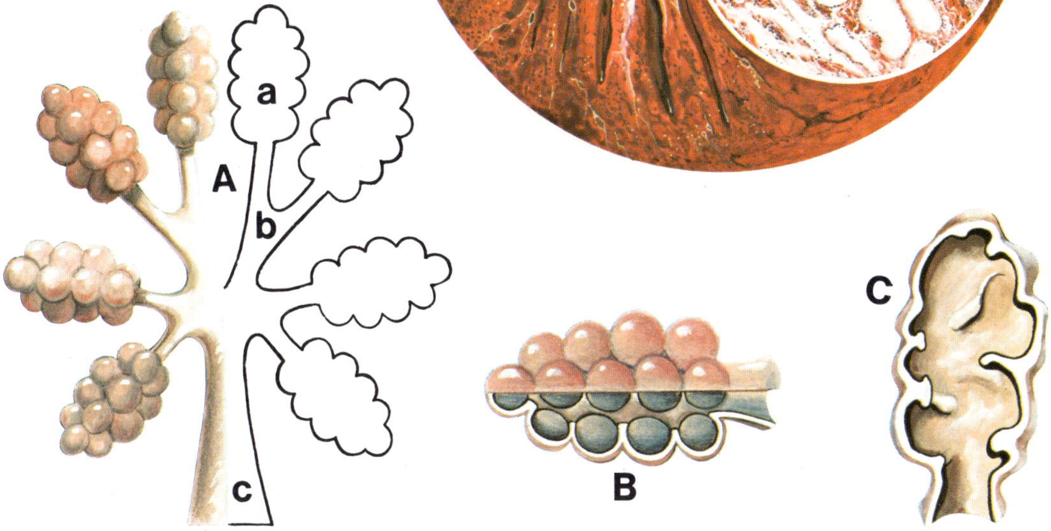

Fig. 51: Chronic catarrhal bronchitis and its consequences in the alveolar region.

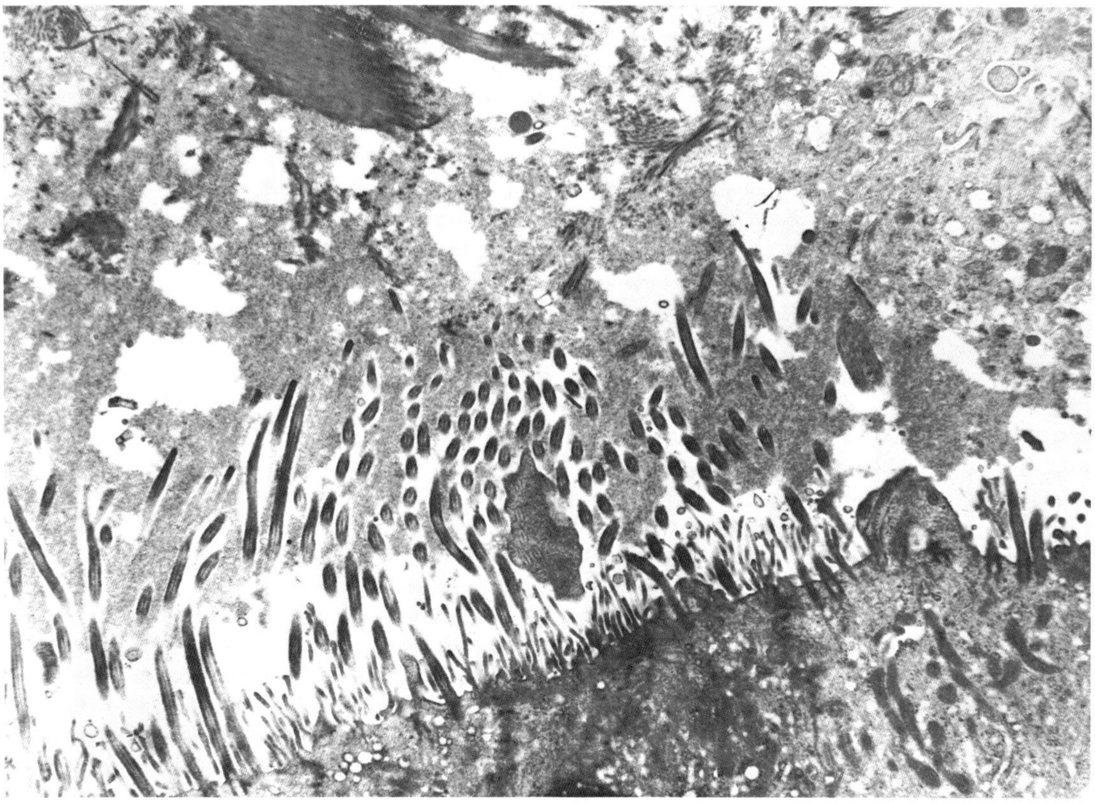

Fig. 52: Chronic bronchitis.
Changes in the secretory layer overlying the bronchial epithelium in chronic bronchitis. The normally uniform sol phase of the secretory layer is lost. Flocculent extensions of increased density of the gel phase extend between the cilia onto the surface of the ciliated cells. The cilia appear trapped in the abnormal secretions which contain fragments of necrotic cells.

TEM
Magnification: 8,200:1

Fig. 53: Chronic bronchitis.
Secretory layer between the cilia and microvilli on the surface of the bronchial epithelium showing increased electron density. Complete loss of the sol phase of the secretory layer. Cilia appear trapped and show clumping (arrows).

TEM
Magnification: 10,000:1

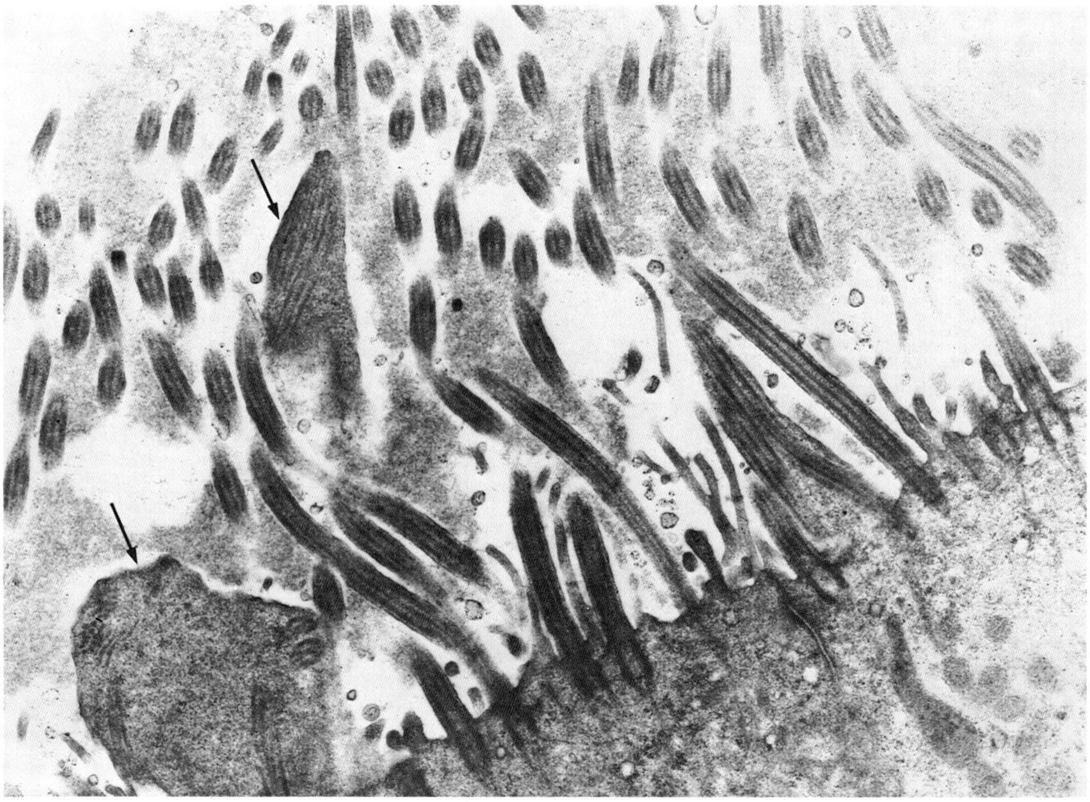

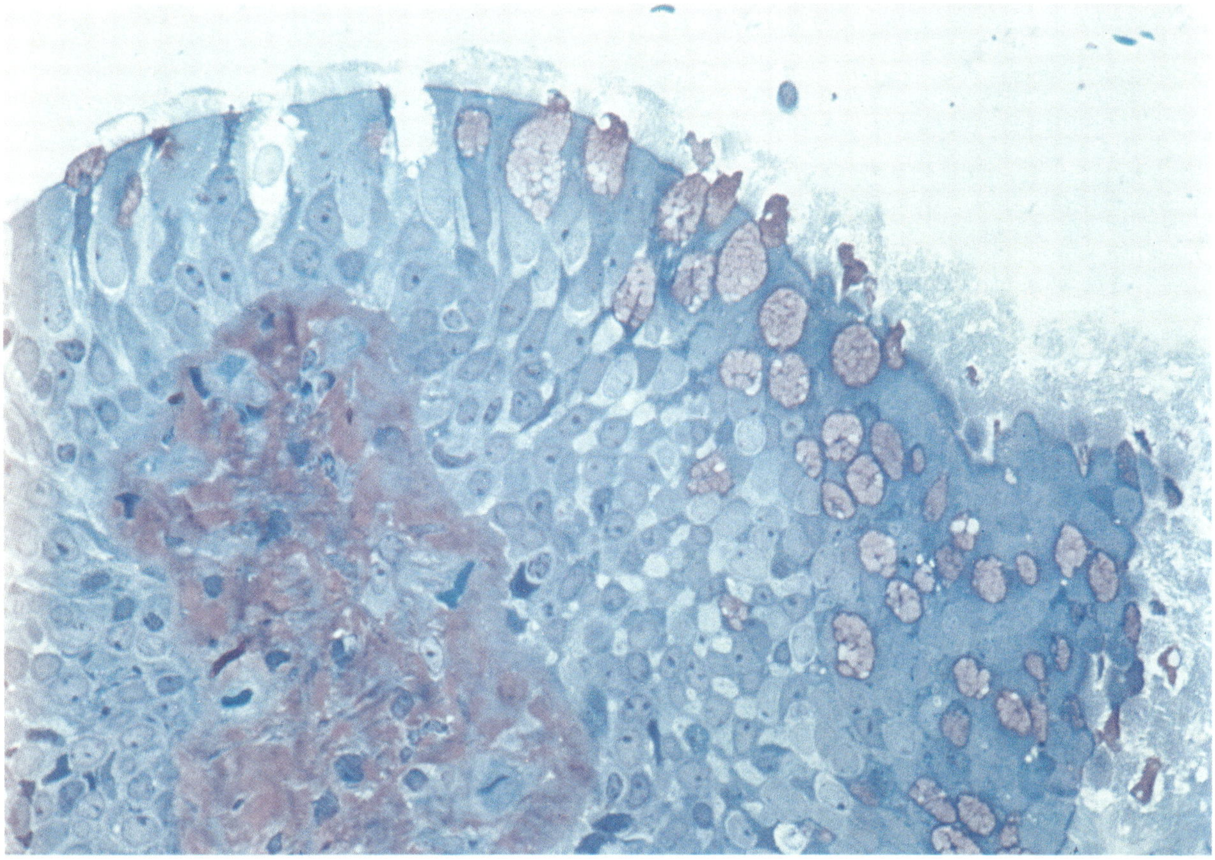

Fig. 54: Chronic bronchitis.
Multiplication of goblet cells in the bronchial epithelium. There are relatively more goblet cells than normal.
LM
Semi-thin section
Stain: Basic fuchsin and methylene blue
Magnification: 1,200:1

Fig. 55: Chronic bronchitis.
Goblet cell hyperplasia in the surface epithelium. The goblet cells are, for the most part, in the same phase of the secretory cycle. Mushroom-like projections of the goblet cells extend far beyond the level of the cilia onto the epithelial surface in the bronchial lumen.

TEM
Magnification: 2,700:1

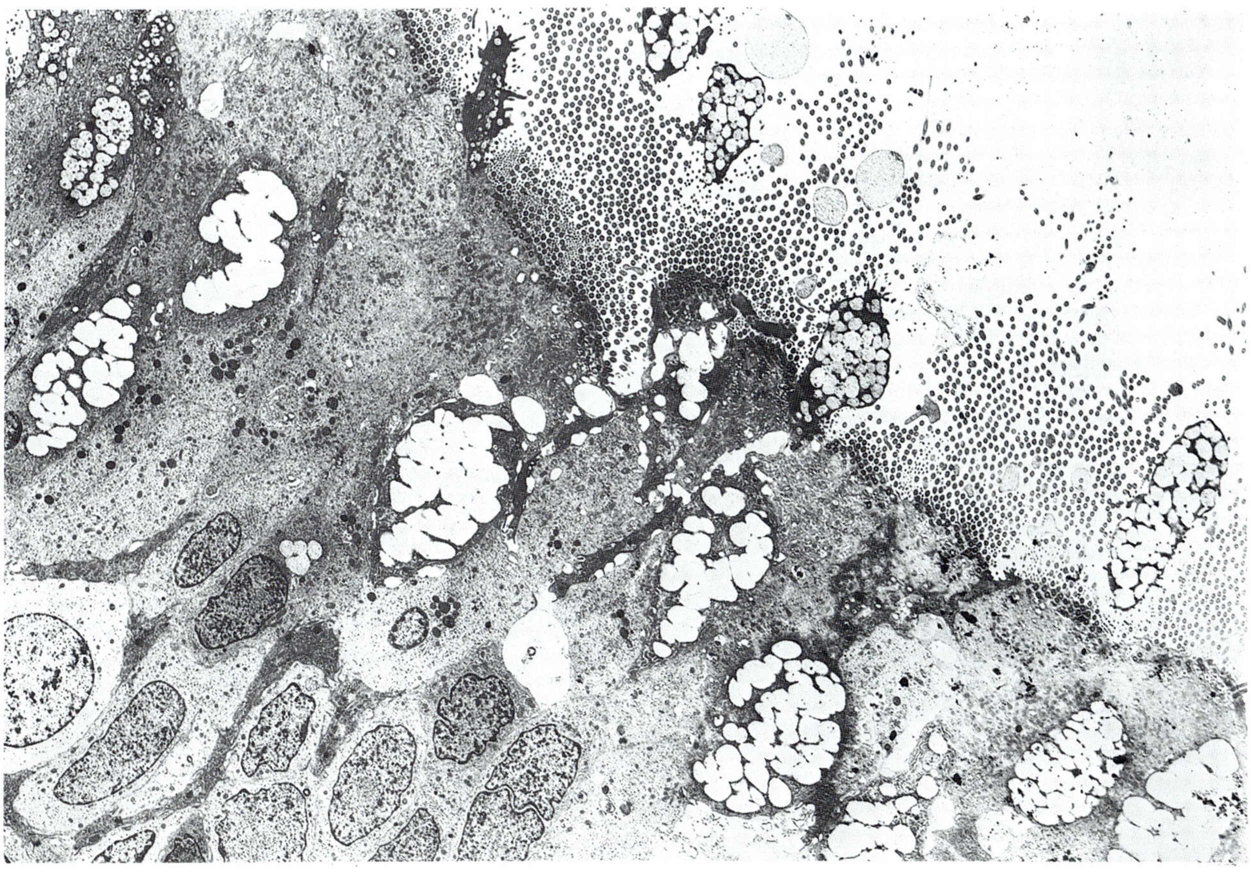

Fig. 56: Chronic bronchitis.
Surface structure of the bronchial epithelium. Increased numbers of goblet cells are seen whose dome-like lumenal projections extend into the bronchial lumen through the ciliated layer.

SEM
Magnification: 5,000:1

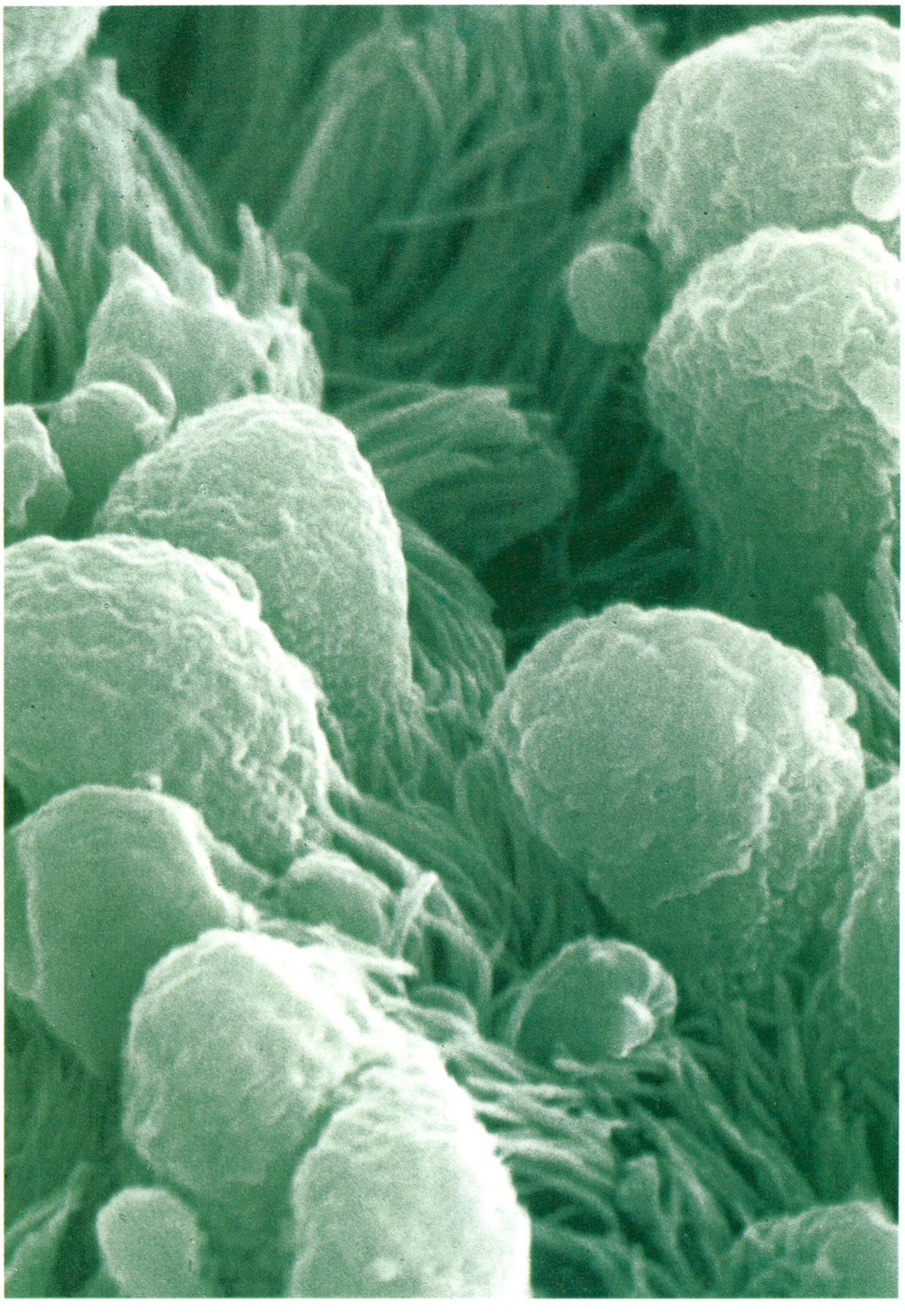

Fig. 57: Chronic bronchitis.
Changes in the basal membrane (BM) of the bronchial epithelium. In the sub-epithelial connective tissue are increased uniform band-like collagen-rich fibres (red).

LM
Semi-thin section
Stain: Basic fuchsin and methylene blue
Magnification: 1,200:1

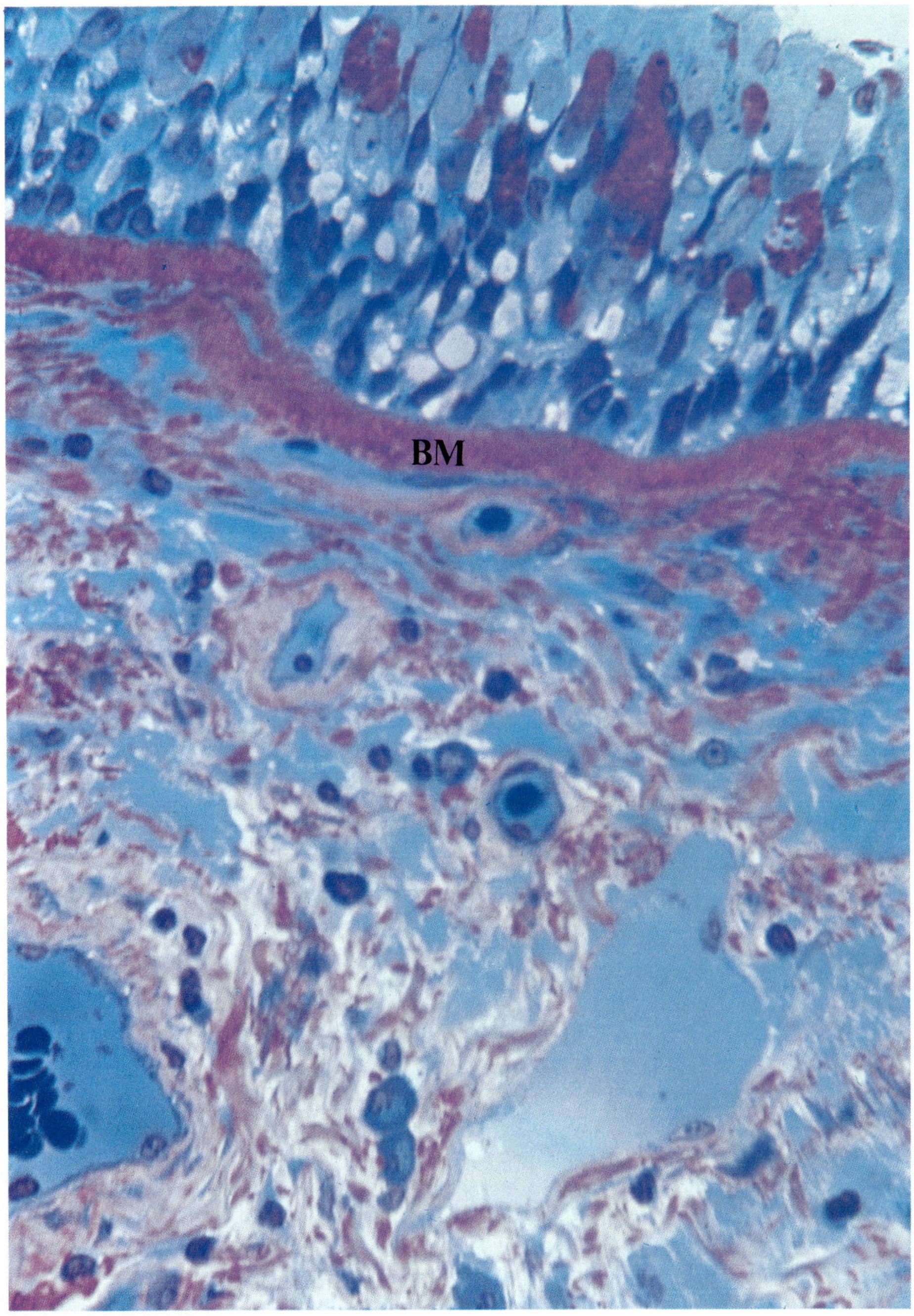

Fig. 58: Chronic bronchitis. Changes in the basal membrane.
Subepithelial zone: Beneath the basal lamella (BL) attached to the undersurface of the epithelium lies a collagen fibre-rich connective tissue zone. This consists of relatively short fibres giving a felt-like appearance. In the deeper layers of this zone are mast cells (M). As a result of these changes, the distance between the epithelium and the subepithelial vascular network is increased.

TEM
Magnification: 2,700:1

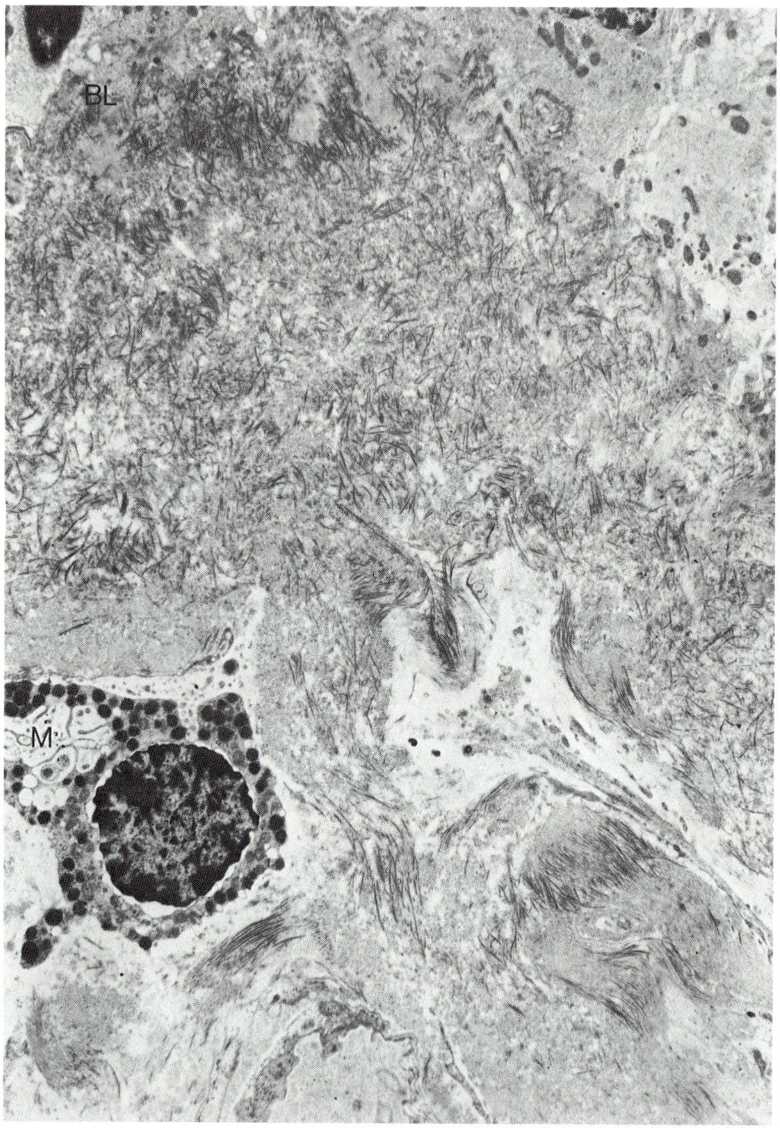

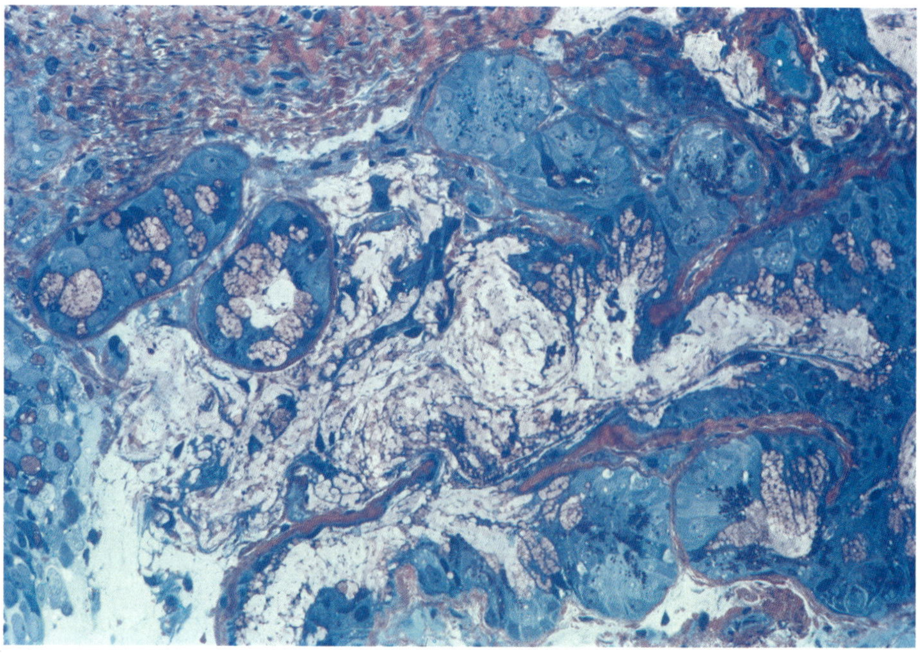

Fig. 59: Chronic bronchitis. Changes in the peribronchial glands.
Mucus transformation of the glandular acini. Cross section shows predominence of the mucous components. The excretory ducts and lumena of the acini are widened and filled with mucus.

LM
Semi-thin section
Stain: Basic fuchsin and methylene blue

Magnification: 850:1

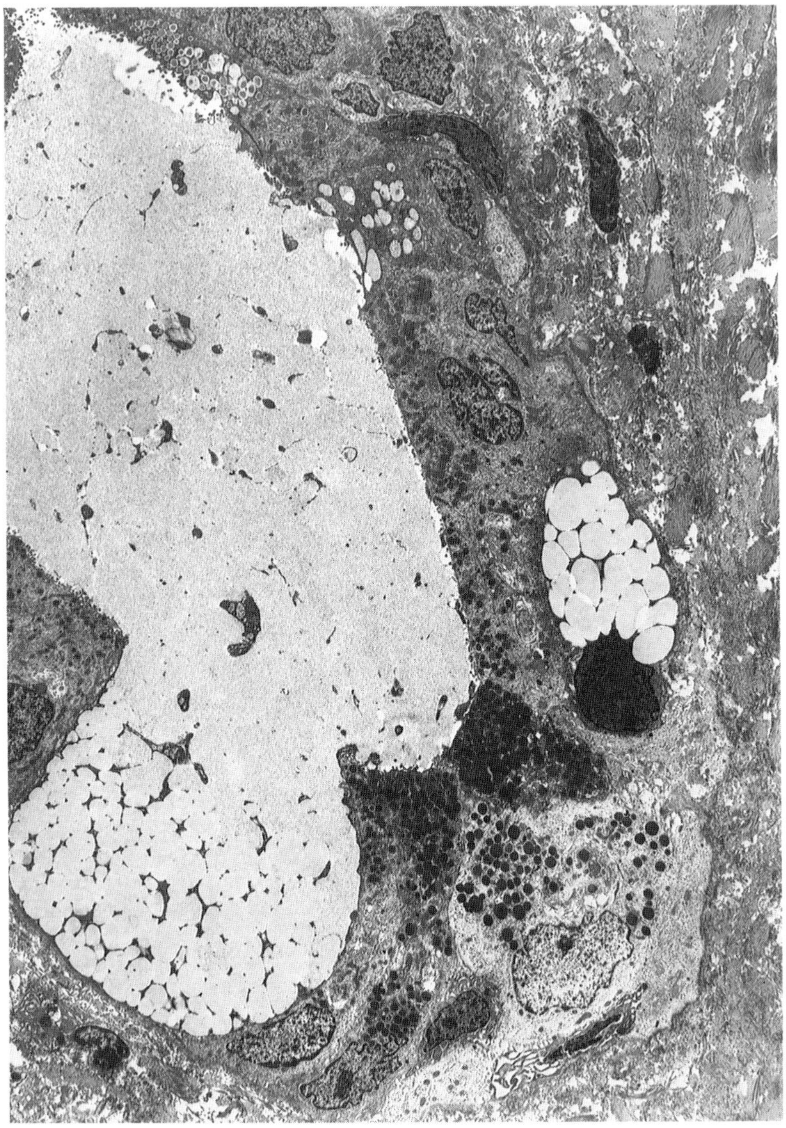

Fig. 60: Chronic bronchitis. Peribronchial gland.
Widened acinus with obstructing mucous plug. The secretion contains cell fragments. Goblet cells in the process of emptying. In the periphery of the section damaged serous epithelial cells.

TEM
Magnification: 3,300:1

Fig. 61: Chronic bronchitis. Densely packed goblet cells in a peribronchial gland.
The majority of goblet cells are in the same phase of secretion formation and discharge. Marked confluence of secretory drops to form large secretory complexes in the cytoplasm of the epithelial cells.

TEM
Magnification: 10,000:1

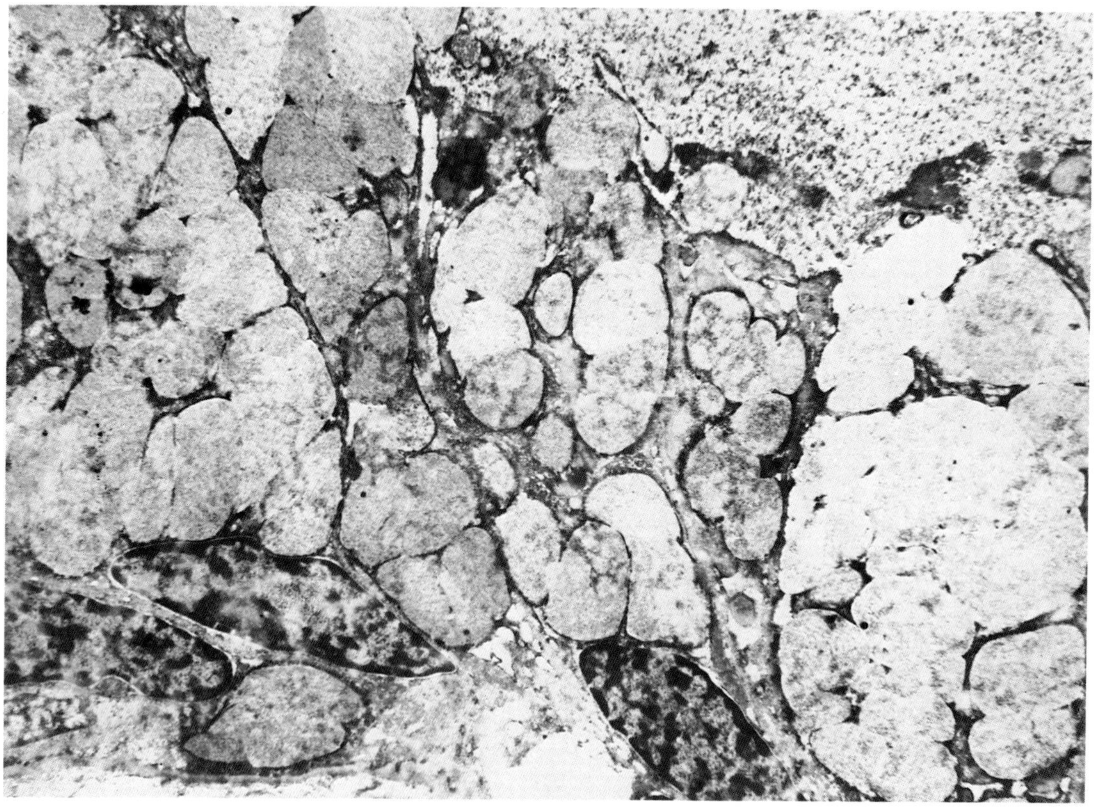

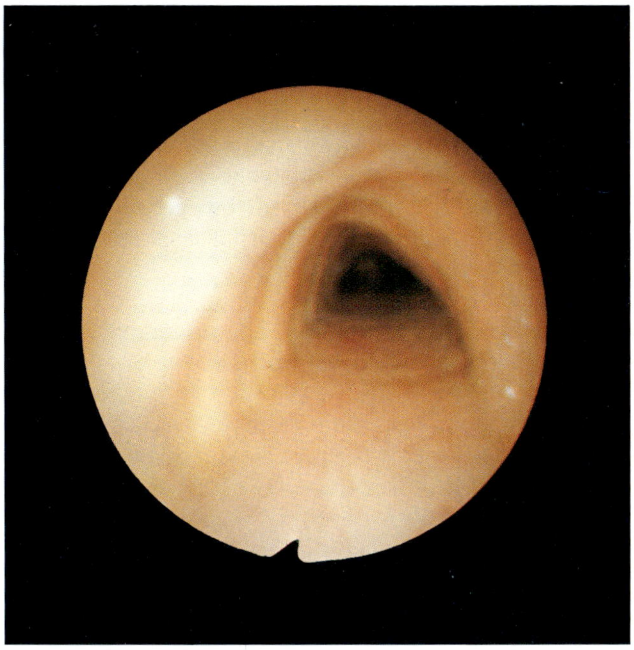

Fig. 62: Chronic bronchitis: Triangular deformation.
This is caused in part by generalized mucosal oedema as well as through softening of tracheal cartilage resulting in this typical deformation and narrowing of the tracheal lumen.

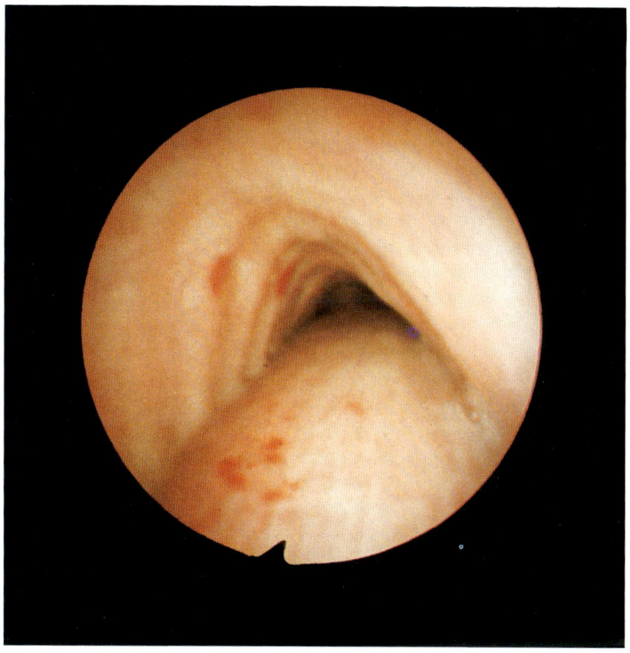

Fig. 63: Chronic bronchitis: Triangular deformation with instability of the pars membranacea (same patient as Fig. 62).
As a result of the loss of elasticity of the tissues of the pars membranacea, the tracheal lumen is narrowed during expiration with increased tracheal obstruction.

Fig. 64: Chronic productive bronchitis.
In addition to mucosal oedema and irregularity, hypersecretion is evident. Because mucociliary transport is impaired, mucus clearance depends almost entirely upon cough.

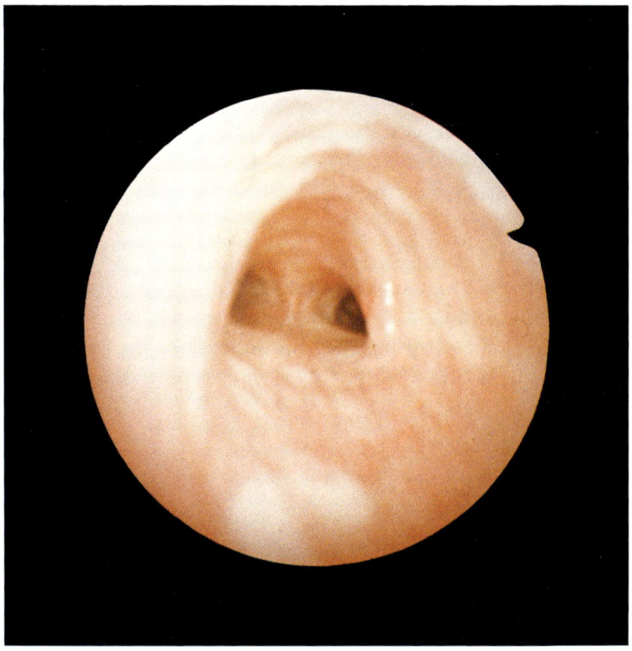

Fig. 65: Chronic productive bronchitis and airway instability (same patient as Fig. 64).
During expiration, herniation of the pars membranacea into the tracheal lumen adds to the narrowing of the trachea caused by mucosal oedema and retained secretions.

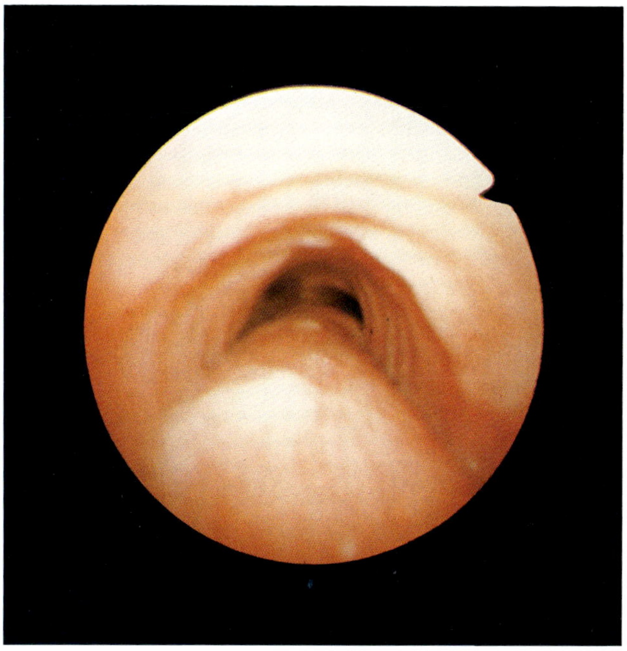

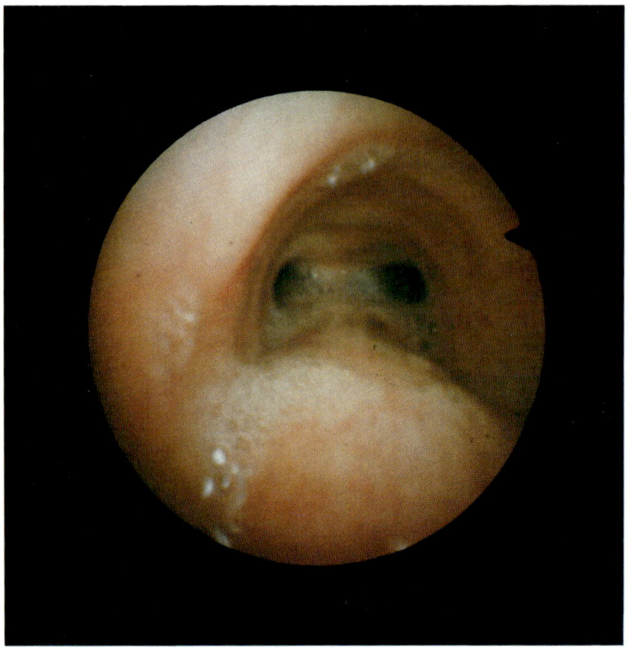

Fig. 66: Chronic productive bronchitis. Exacerbation.
As a result of superinfection, increased hypersecretion and inflammatory exudate leads to increased airways obstruction. This contributes to alveolar hypoventilation resulting in CO_2 retention and hypoxaemia, characteristic of respiratory failure.

Fig. 67: Chronic productive bronchitis. Exacerbation. Therapeutic lavage.
The bronchus on the left is now patent, while secretions still partially occlude that on the right.

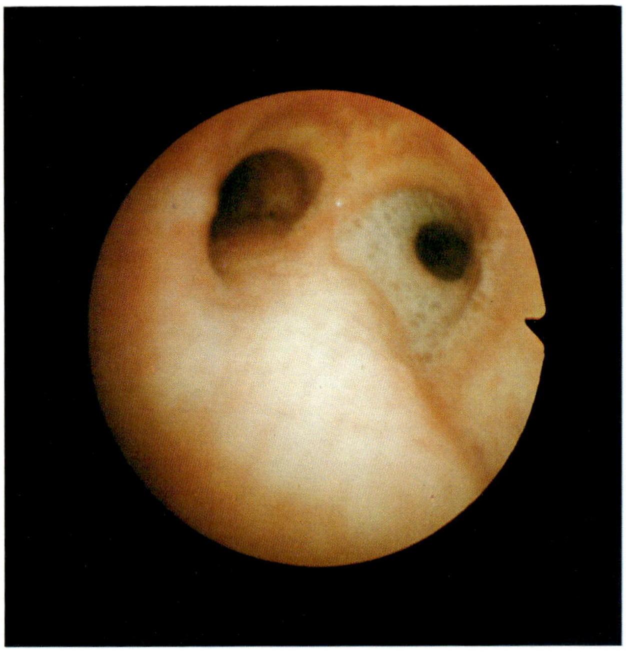

3.3.2. Chronic Intramural Bronchitis

This condition is characterized by a more or less marked and irregularly distributed inflammatory cell reaction in the subepithelial connective tissue as demonstrated in biopsy and postmortem specimens. The cellular infiltrates may vary in composition, but consist predominantly of lymphocytes and plasma cells as well as a variable number of neutrophils. Acute bronchitic exacerbations are superimposed upon the chronic low grade inflammatory reaction. The inflammatory infiltrate penetrates the surface epithelium.

These exacerbations result from bacterial superinfection, usually by mixed organisms. Mucosal necrosis with ulcerations of varying depth may occur with subsequent scarring and stenosis resulting in obliteration of the bronchial lumen. Squamous metaplasia may be associated with the scarring, particularly if the surface epithelium has been seriously injured. During acute exacerbations, alveolar ventilation is further reduced because of mucous plugging associated with increased mucus production and the presence of purulent secretions. The frequency of acute exacerbations increases with the duration of the disease.

The cause of the exacerbations is not always clear. Frequently, bacterial infections due to Haemophilus influenza, Diplococcus pneumoniae or Pseudomonas aeruginosa may occur but cultures may reveal only "normal flora". Reinfection of the lower respiratory tract from infected sinuses has been described and in recent years intermittent, subtle aspiration of refluxed gastric contents has been implicated as a possible cause.

Because of the patchy nature of the process in the airway, isolated biopsies may be of little value for describing the morphological changes in the entire airway. Thus, several biopsies from various parts of the airway showing similar changes should be obtained, before a valid conclusion can be drawn about the extent and severity of the disease process. In the hyperaemic, oedematous mucosa, zones of polypoid proliferation may be seen. There is evidence of increased mucus production. The small and medium sized bronchi are greatly narrowed by mucosal oedema, excessive and frequently infected secretions and bronchospasm. Between the thickened and prominent submucosal elastic fibres, the mucosa shows furrowing, giving the mucosal surface an irregular rope ladder-like appearance.

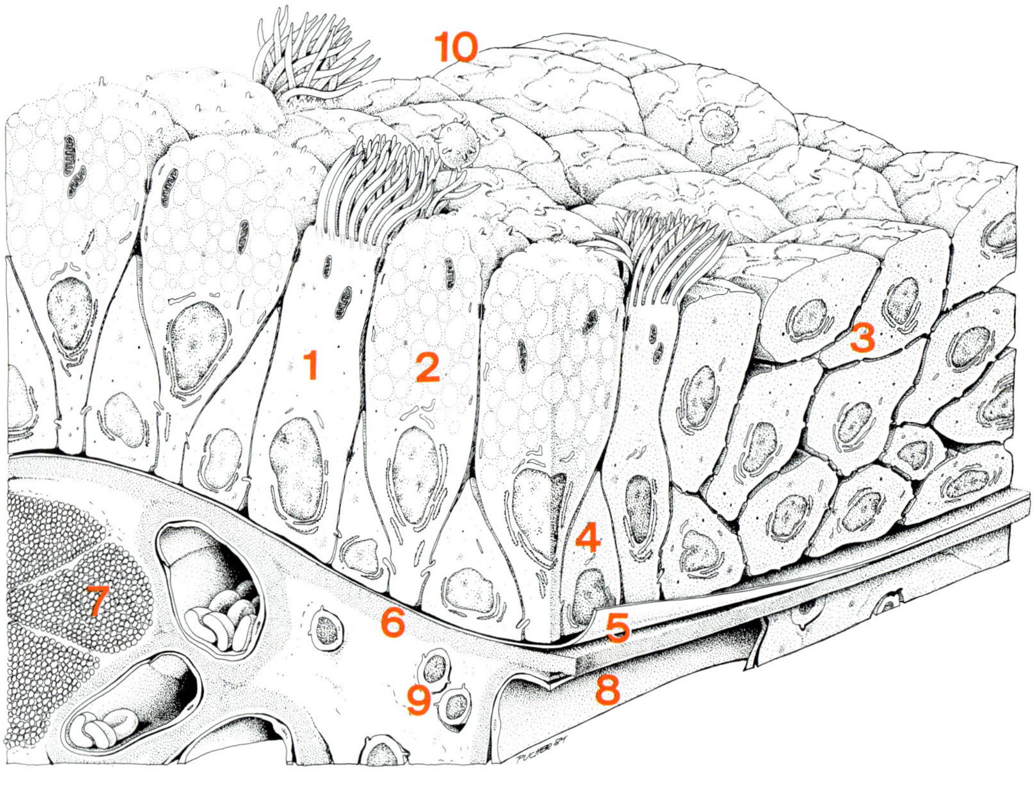

Fig. 68: Chronic bronchitis. Three-dimensional diagram of changes in the surface layer of the bronchial mucosa.

1: ciliated cells
2: goblet cells
3: irregularly arranged squamous metaplasia
4: basal cells of the bronchial epithelium
5: basal lamella of the bronchial epithelium
6: subepithelial clearly widened fibrous zone
7: smooth muscle
8: vessels of the bronchial wall
9: slight inflammatory cell infiltration of the submucosa
10: irregularly distributed secretions on the mucosal surface

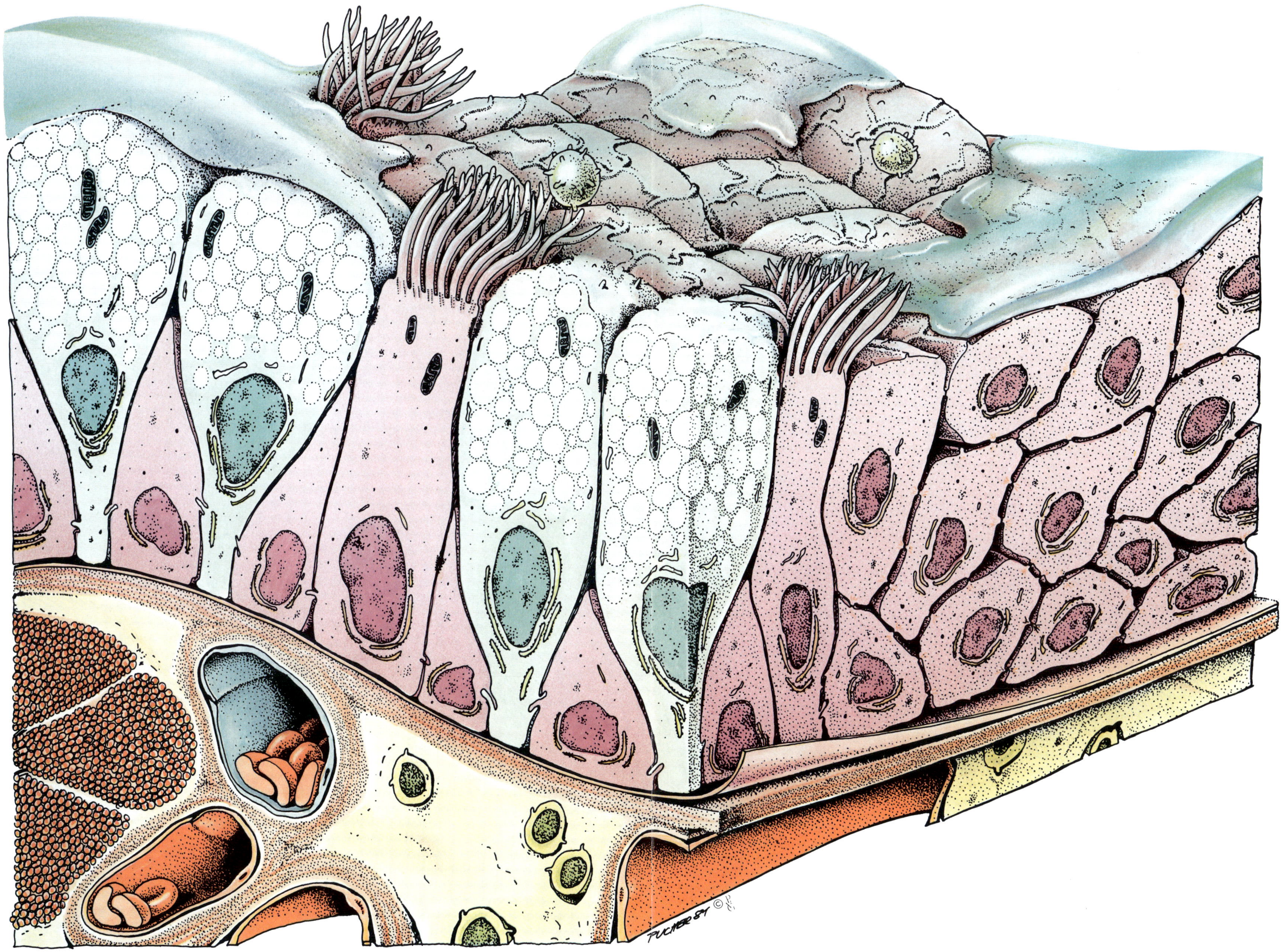
PUCHER 84 ©

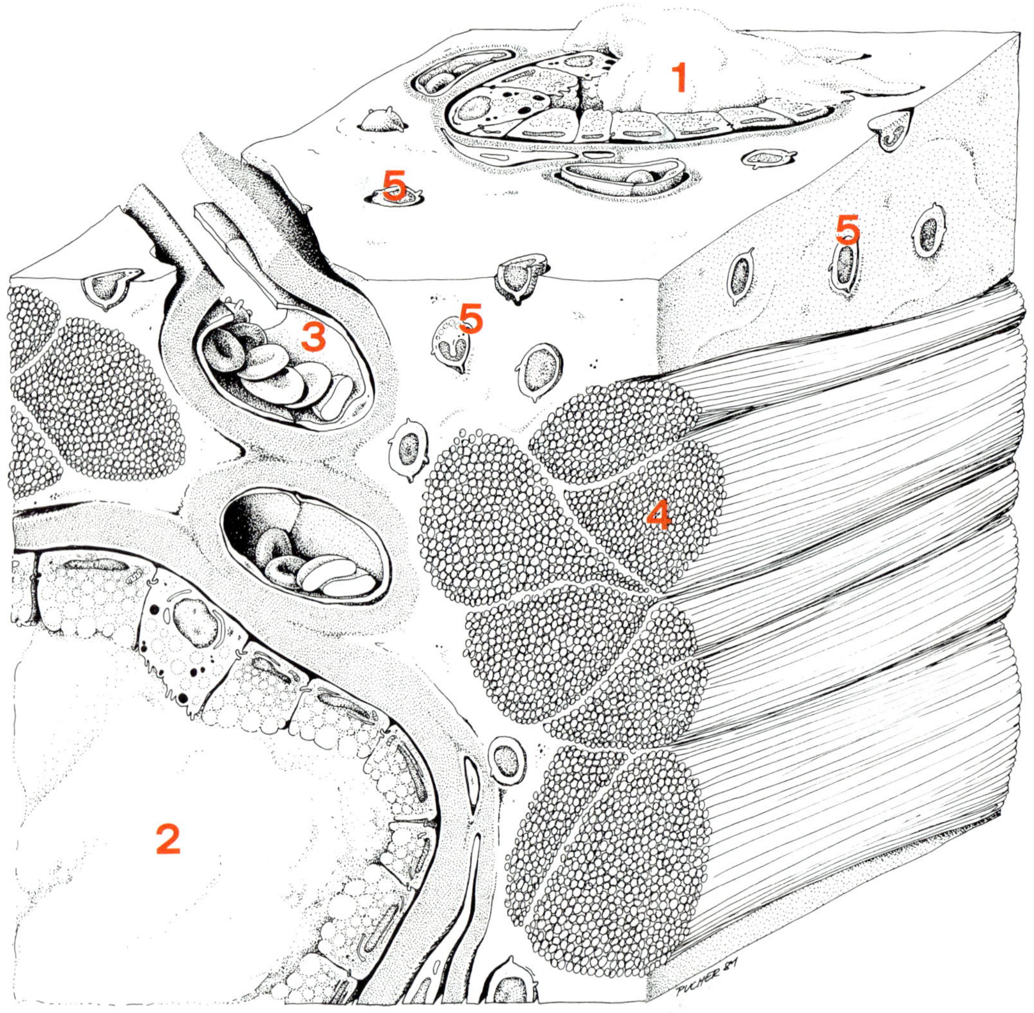

Fig. 69: Chronic bronchitis. Alterations in the deeper layers of the bronchial wall.

1: mucous plug in a dilated excretory duct of a peribronchial gland
2: mucous transformation in the peribronchial gland with distension of the acinar lumen containing accumulated tenacious secretions
3: submucosal vessels with perivascular fibrous tissue
4: smooth muscle
5: sparse inflammatory cell infiltration of the submucosa

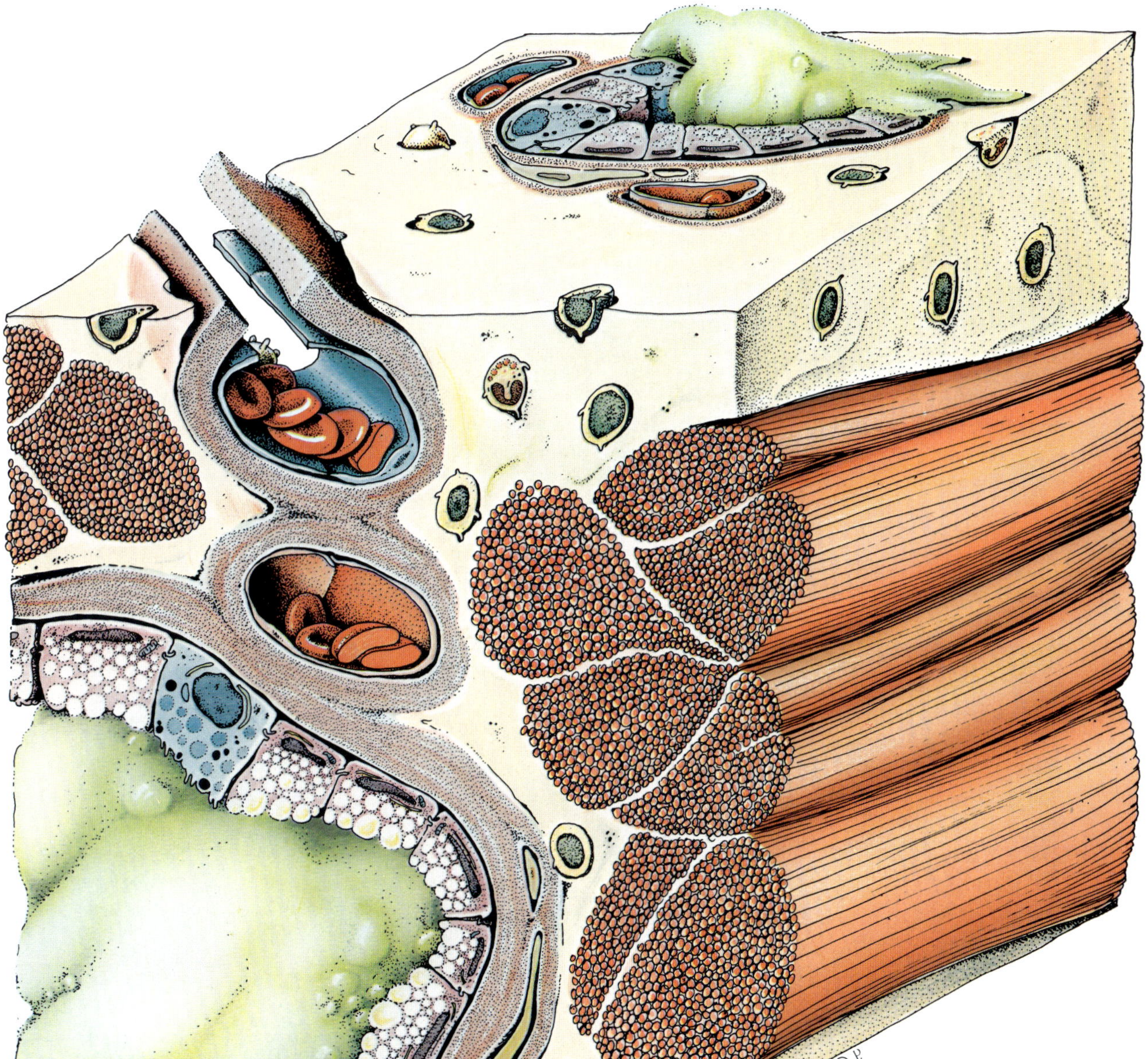

3.3.3. Hypertrophic Bronchitis

Recurring mainly bacterial infections of the bronchial mucosa may lead to a polypoid thickening and furrowing. Lymph follicles develop in the deeper layers of the submucosa and extend to the adventitia. Large patches of squamous metaplasia are commonly seen. This hypertrophic type of inflammation is seen in large bronchi, particularly in bronchiectasis. In late stages, the mucosal hypertrophy may change to atrophy. In the thickened velvety mucosa are seen zones of polypoid epithelial proliferation. The epithelium produces increased secretions. The medium and small bronchi are narrowed as a result of mucosal oedema, secretion and inflammatory exudate. Between the thickened raised elastic fibre bundles of the submucosa, the mucosa may show slight herniation resulting in an irregular rope ladder-like appearance of the inner surface of the bronchial wall.

Fig. 70: Chronic bronchitis. Loss of cilia in the surface epithelium.
Cilia remain only on occasional cells. The cell boundaries of the epithelial cells are slightly raised outlining the mosaic-like epithelial structure.

SEM
Magnification: 1,200:1

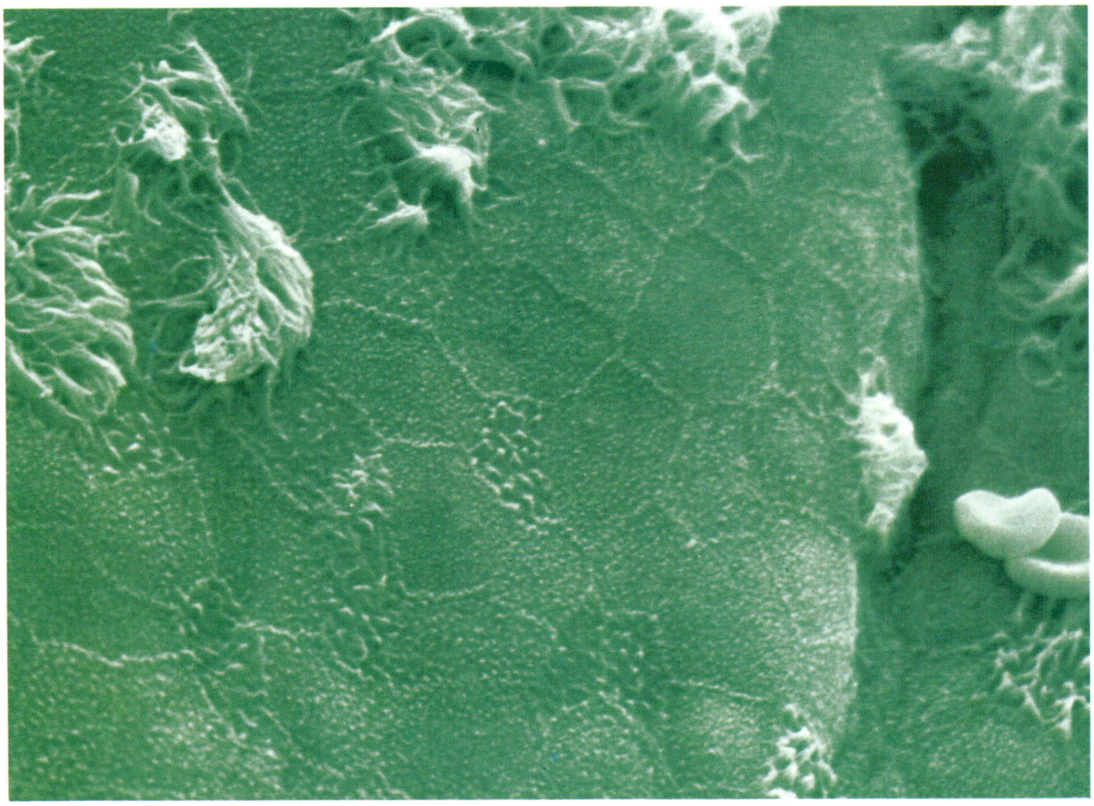

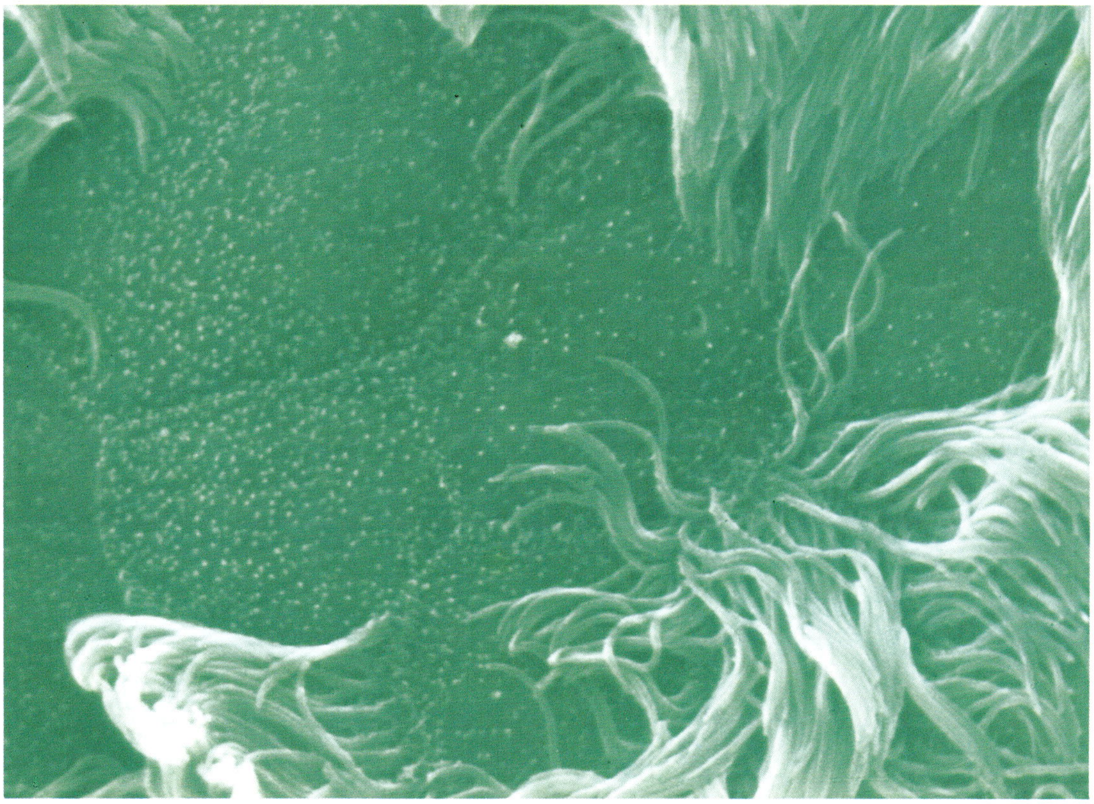

Fig. 71: Chronic bronchitis. Patches of surface epithelium have been denuded of cilia and show uniformly distributed microvilli. The concentration of microvilli is greater along cell boundaries. Some cells show relatively well maintained ciliary structure.

SEM
Magnification: 5,000:1

Fig. 72: Chronic bronchitis. The surface epithelium shows loss of cilia in large areas. The surface of the epithelial cells has a velvety appearance because of irregularly distributed microvilli. Individual inflammatory cells are seen lying along the epithelial surface.

SEM
Magnification: 920:1

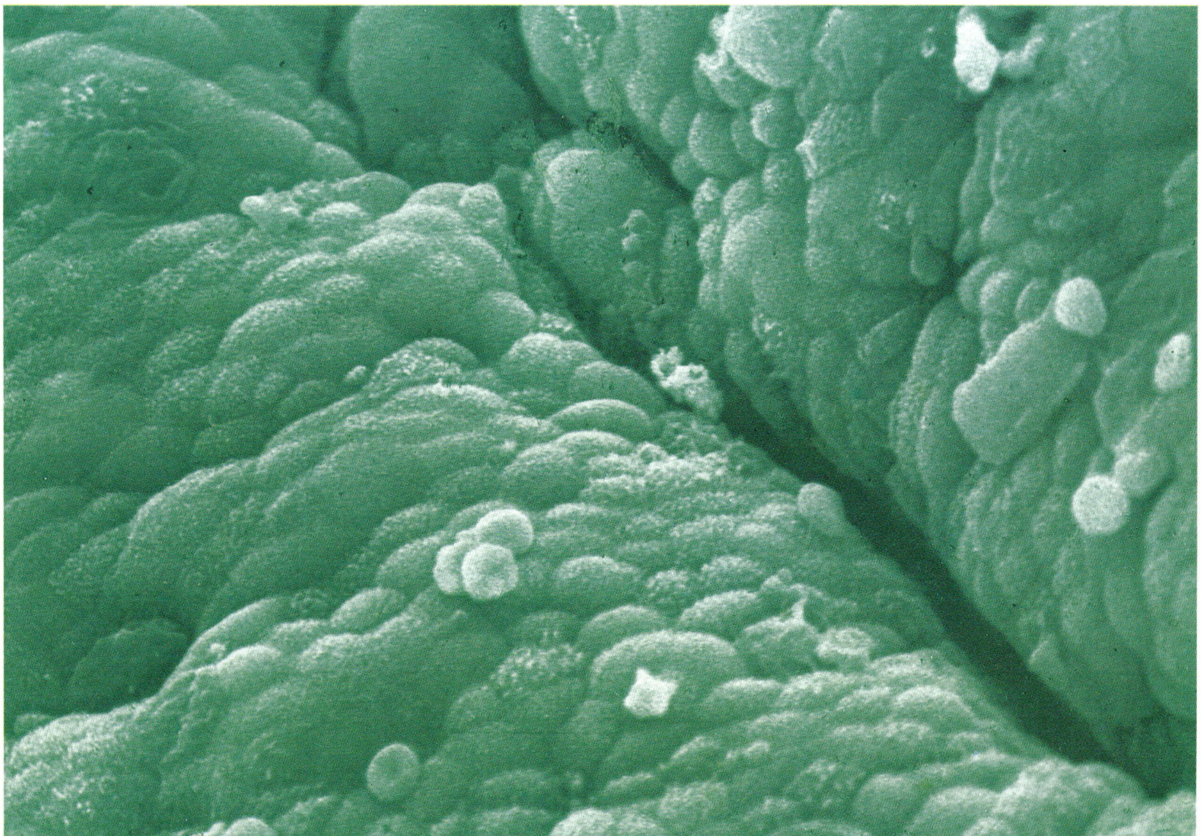

3.3.4. Chronic Destructive Bronchitis

As a result of increasing scarring of the submucosa, various elements of the bronchial wall disappear. The peribronchial glands are enveloped by scar tissue and decrease in number. The supporting cartilage may also be affected and may even disintegrate. The inflammatory infiltrate may vary in severity and composition. It consists mainly of lymphocytes and plasma cells, except during obvious bacterial infections when typical polymorphonuclear leukocytes are evident. The number and density of collagen fibres increase markedly, particularly in the submucosa. This is seen as a thickening of the basement membrane on light micoscopy. Especially with this type of bronchitis, patches of mucosa are seen in which the ciliated epithelium is replaced by squamous metaplasia. Such changes may be irreversible.

The morphological appearance predicts severe dysfunction which is usually found in this type of chronic bronchitis. The relatively fixed severe airways obstruction doubtlessly results from a combination of retained secretions because of impaired mucociliary transport, mucosal oedema resulting from chronic inflammation and pe-

Fig. 73: Chronic bronchitis. Extensive squamous metaplasia of the surface epithelium.
There is loss of the well organized pseudostratified squamous bronchial epithelium. Within the squamous epithelium is a uniform layer with differentiation of spindle cells. The subepithelial connective tissue zone contains a relatively sparse inflammatory cell infiltrate.

LM
Stain: Basic fuchsin and methylene blue
Magnification: 1,240:1

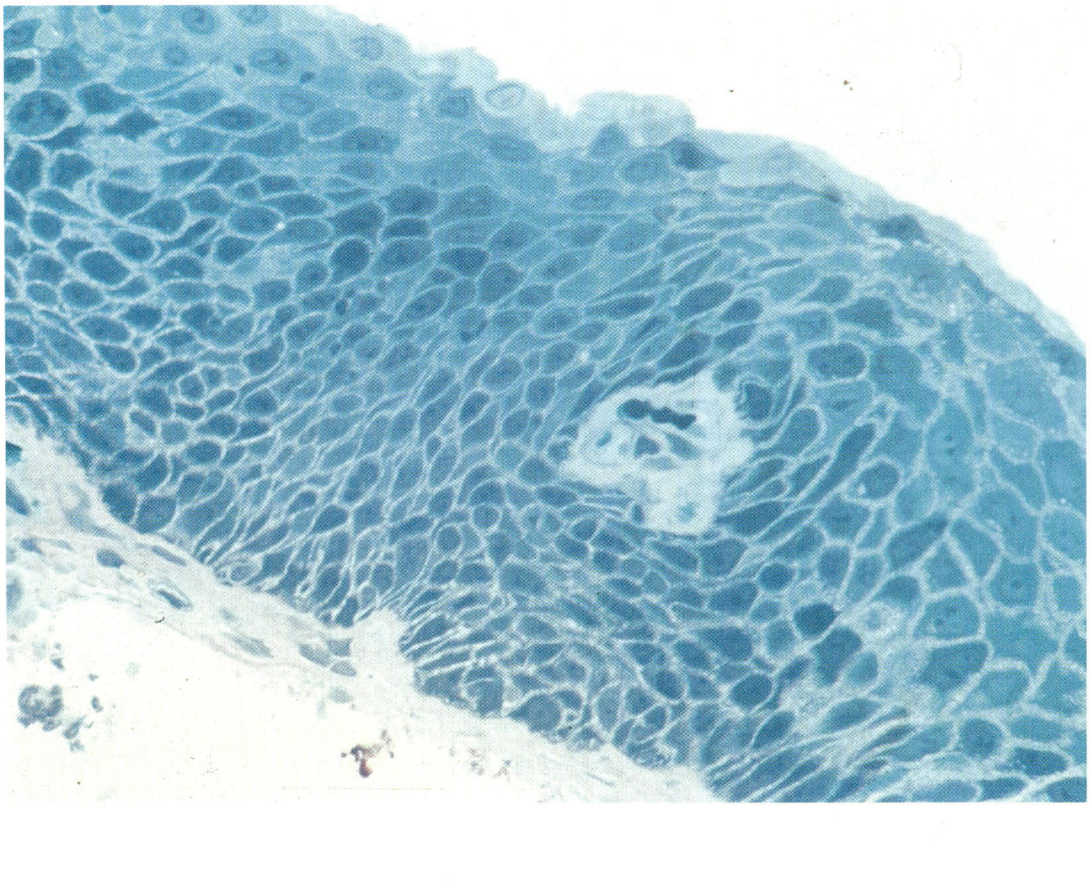

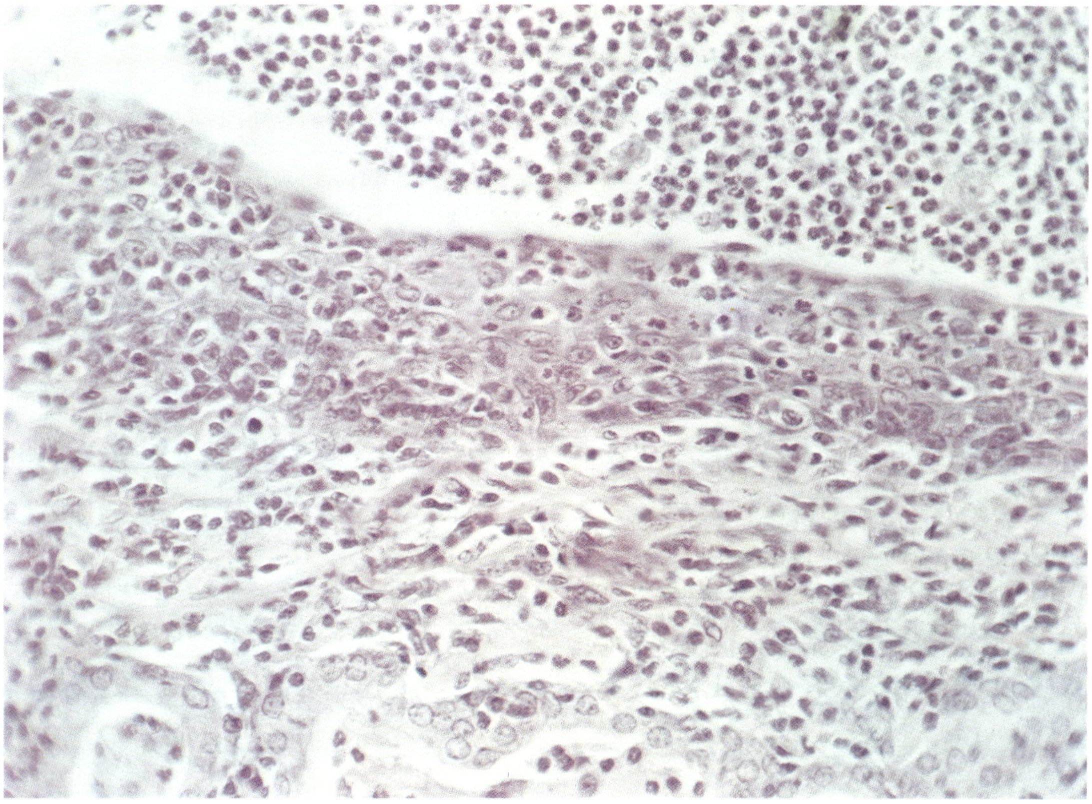

Fig. 74: Chronic bronchitis. Acute exacerbation. Many leukocytes are seen in the subepithelial connective tissue in the metaplastic squamous epithelium of the bronchial surface and in the bronchial lumen. As a result of leukocyte migration in the epithelium there is marked loosening of epithelial junctions.

LM
Stain: Hematoxylin-eosin
Magnification: 480:1

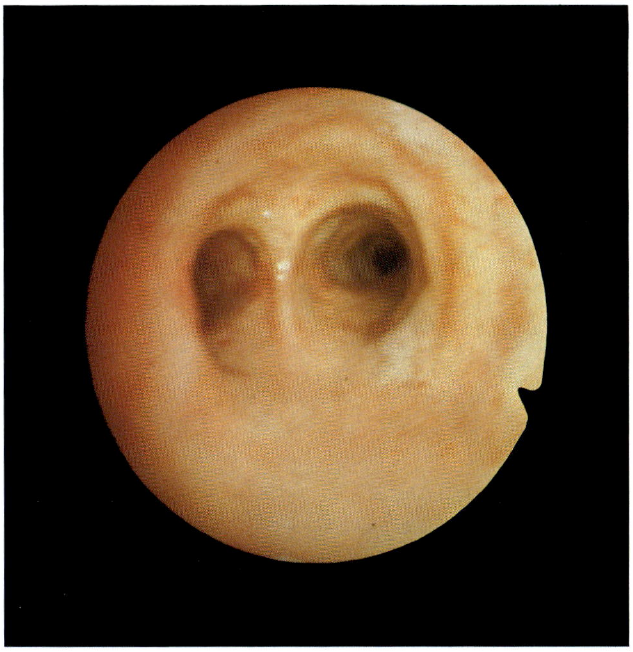

Fig. 75: Chronic atrophic bronchitis. The mucosa appears pale. The carina is very thin and airway instability may be very marked.

ribronchial fibrosis with eventual stenosis, particularly in medium and small bronchioles. More peripheral airways may be partially or completed occluded by inflammatory exudate. The mucosa may bulge between the elastic fibres of the submucosa, which are thickened and prominent, so that the inner surface of the bronchial wall takes on a rope ladder-like appearance.

3.3.5. Peribronchitis

In severe and longstanding intramural and destructive bronchitis, inflammatory changes may spread to the peribronchial tissues resulting in circumferential scars. The inflammatory reaction extends to some extent into the adjacent pulmonary tissue.

Fig. 76: Chronic bronchitis. Squamous metaplasia.
The cell boundaries are clearly seen on the surface because they are slightly raised. The surface epithelium is irregular because of the partly amorphous, partly corrugated surface structure of individual epithelial cells. Occasional inflammatory cells are seen on the surface (arrows).

SEM
Magnification: 4,200:1

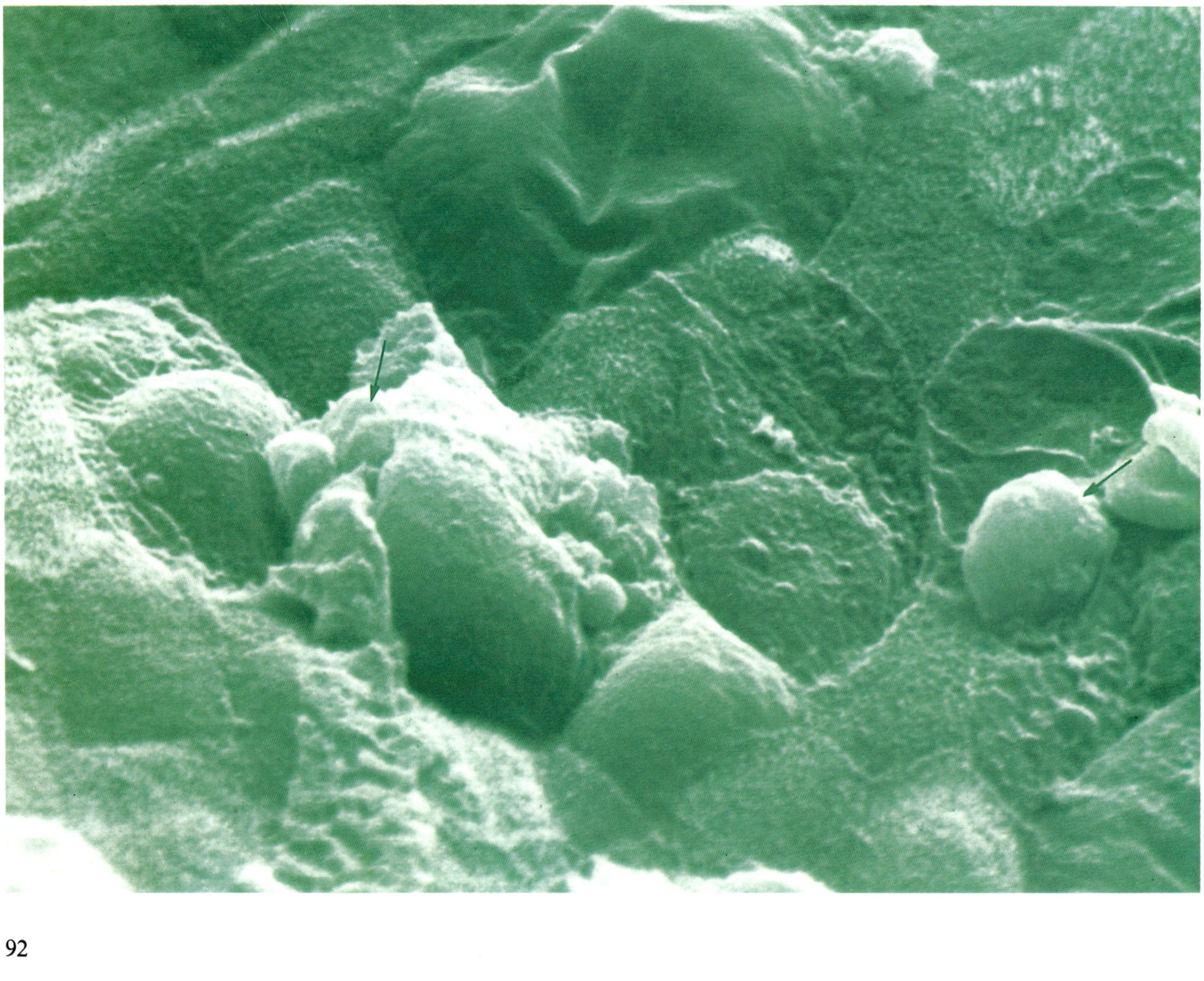

3.4. Specific Inflammatory Responses of the Bronchial Mucosa

Tuberculosis:
In this condition, characteristic granulation tissue may develop in the bronchial mucosa. It may involve the airways from the lumen, or by haematogenous or lymphogenous spread. In cavitary tuberculosis, the inflammatory reaction is usually limited to the supplying bronchus. Enlarged hilar lymph nodes may, in conditions such as tuberculosis, silico-tuberculosis, silicosis and sarcoidosis, compress the bronchial wall resulting in compression and distortion of the airways. Recurring post-obstructive infections may lead to chronic bronchitis and bronchiectasis. Such changes have been called bronchitis deformans.

Sarcoidosis:
While hilar lymphadenopathy and parenchymal granulomas are most commonly seen, about 70% of patients with clinical sarcoidosis may, at bronchial biopsy, show the pathological features of non-caseating granulomas. Such patients may present with bronchitis and usually respond to steroid therapy.

Fig. 77: Sarcoidosis. Bronchial wall.
Multiple epithelioid cell granulomas without central necrosis from the bronchial wall of a biopsy specimen. The bronchial epithelium over the granulomas is intact. Around the granulomas is a circumferential collagen fibre zone.

LM
Stain: van Gieson
Magnification: 420:1

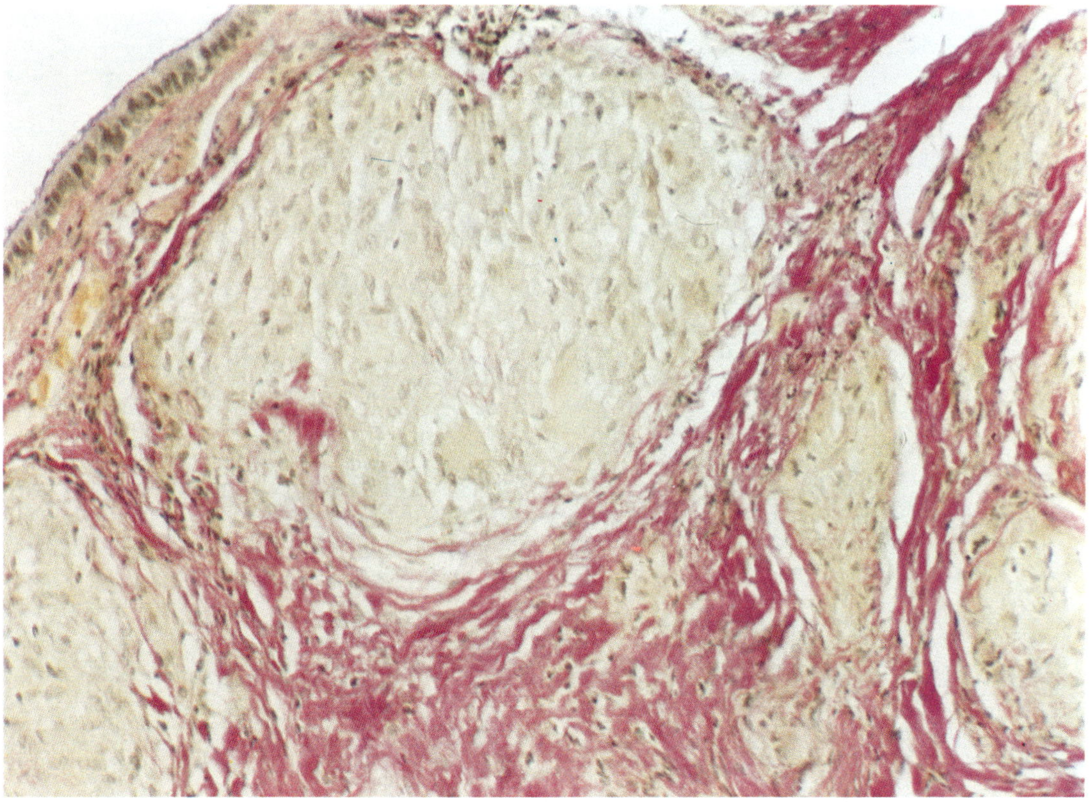

Fig. 78: Sarcoidosis. Bronchial wall granuloma from a biopsy specimen. The granuloma contains a Langhans giant cell showing an asteroid body.

LM
Semi-thin section
Stain: Basic fuchsin and methylene blue
Magnification: 1,200:1

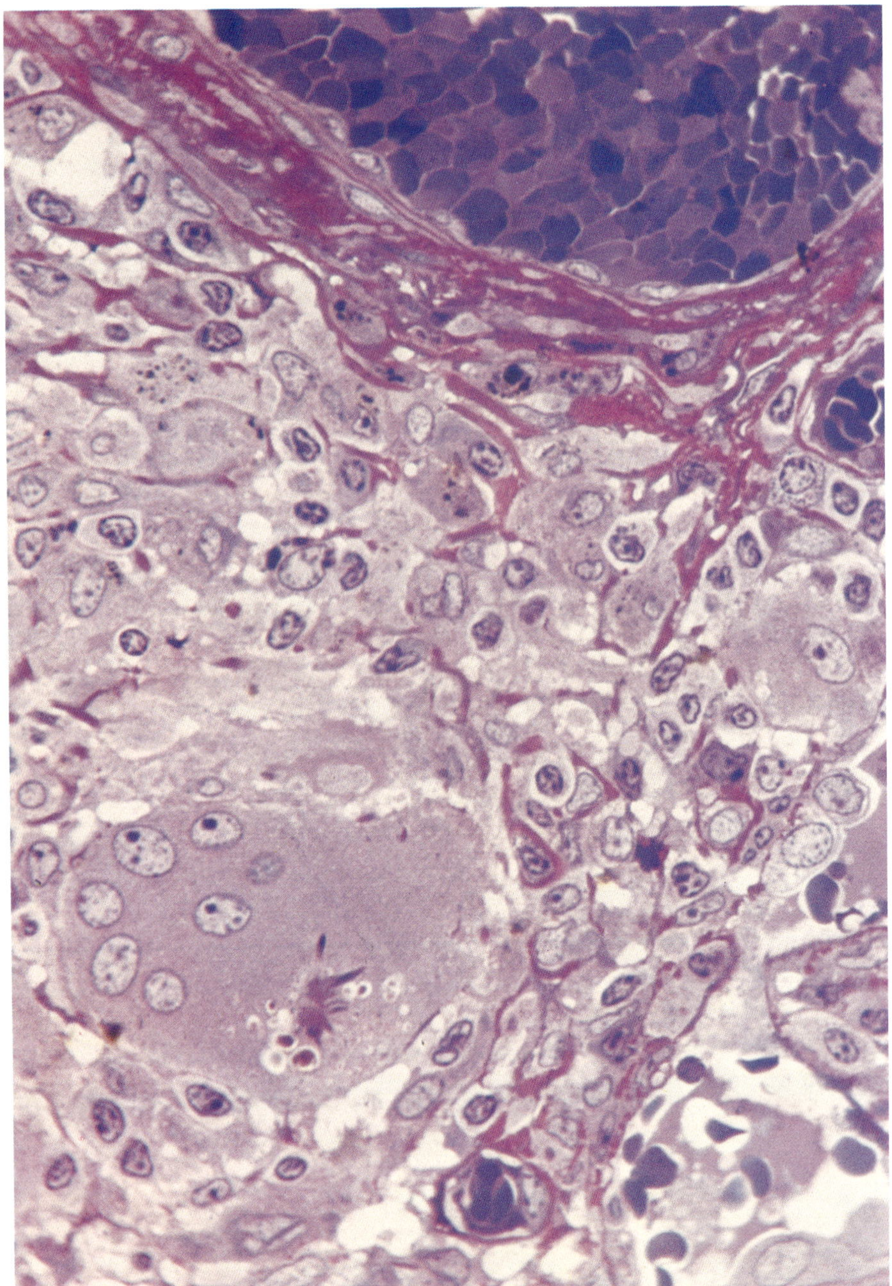

3.5. Nonspecific Associated Bronchial Wall Reactions in Pulmonary Tuberculosis

Pulmonary tuberculosis is frequently associated with a nonspecific inflammatory reaction of the tracheobronchial tree without evidence of typical caseating granulomas. Such bronchitis might accout for severe persistent cough and assist dissemination of the tubercle bacillus throughout the airway particularly into the mucosa and the peribronchial gland ducts. The morphological appearance of these nonspecific changes of the bronchial wall vary only with respect to their severity, but otherwise show an almost identical picture to that of chronic catarrhal bronchitis. The changes affect mainly the squamous epithelium and the peribronchial glands. The surface epithelium shows many goblet cells in various stages of the secretory cycle. Squamous metaplasia is commonly seen. The basement membrane may show 6-8 fold hypertrophy. Adjacent to the basal cell layer runs a thin uninterrupted basement membrane of approximately 700 A. It is, in turn, joined by a network of fine, densely packed collagenous and reticular fibres. The microvilli of the ciliated cells are markedly decreased suggesting a high cell turnover rate. Mitochondria, important suppliers of energy to the ciliated cells, are greatly decreased in number and show morphological changes.

The mucous components of the peribronchial glands show accelerated formation of secretion and for the most part are in an advanced stage of the secretory cycle. Discharge of excessive volumes of secretion may be associated with cell necrosis, which may in turn result in extensive defects in the epithelial lining of the glandular acini. Because the viscous secretions cannot be excreted as fast as they are produced, cystic dilatation of the acinar and excretory duct system may result. Mucous transformation of the peribronchial glands develops as an expression of disordered secretion. The inflammatory cell reaction in the glandular stroma is relatively sparse and characterized mainly by accumulation of lymphocytes and plasma cells. With time, vascular changes may also occur. Around the vessels, several layers of basal lamellae surrounded by circumferentially arranged collagen fibres develop. The peribronchial gland acini are also surrounded by a concentric fibrous zone. As a result of the compression of glandular elements and vessels by increasing fibrosis, the nutrition of the tissues becomes increasingly compromised, resulting in glandular atrophy.

Vigourous therapy directed at the inflammatory reaction, at least in the initial stages of the disorder, may assist in re-establishing the normal secretory activity of the mucosa. As a result, the serous components of the glandular acini increase and their cells show increased activity. Presumably, because of the decreased inflammation and increased clearance of secretions from the excretory ducts, regeneration of a normal epithelium occurs. Following restoration of normal secretory function of the mucosa, there is also an increase in the microvilli of the ciliated cells. As a result of the increased activity of the serous components of the glands as well as restoration of a normal ciliated epithelium, mucociliary transport may be restored.

3.6. Bronchial Asthma

Bronchial asthma is characterized by episodic breathlessness, alternating with periods of relative normality, either spontaneously or as result of therapy. During exacerbations, dilatation of peripheral airways and alveoli occurs, resulting in gas trapping secondary to airways obstruction. The airways obstruction is the result of a combination of bronchospasm, mucosal oedema and retained secretions. During remissions, virtually all of the changes may regress. Variable dyspnea associated with so-called asthmatic bronchitis in adults or bronchiolitis in children should be regarded as asthma equivalents.

Extrinsic allergic or atopic asthma results from an immediate (type I) reaction affecting the bronchial mucosa, frequently caused by well recognized, usually inhaled, antigens. Rarely, antigens may enter via the gastrointestinal tract or parenterally. The reaction involves IgE which occupies receptors on the surface of the target cells - mast cells and basophils. As a result of the antigen-antibody reaction, the affected cells degranulate and release mediators including histamine, slow-reacting substance (SRS-A, bradykinin), serotonin, etc., which act directly on various components of the bronchial mucosa.

During an asthmatic attack, the appearance of the bronchial mucosa is characterized by bronchoconstriction, excessive amounts of abnormal secretions, increased numbers of goblet cells in the bronchial epithelium, mucous transformation of the peribronchial glands and mucosal inflammatory changes with oedema and eosinophilia.

Immediately following the allergic reaction in the bronchial mucosa, bronchoconstriction occurs as a re

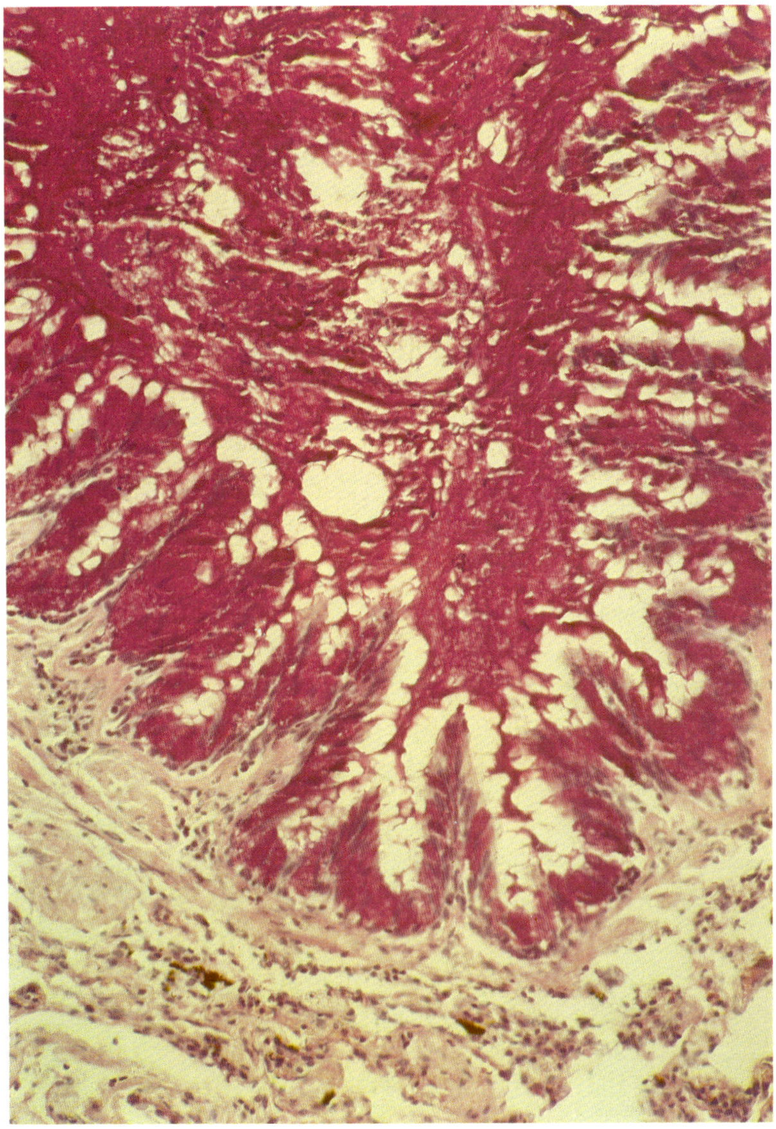

Fig. 79: Bronchial asthma. Bronchial cross section.
Because of smooth contraction in the bronchial wall there is a star-shaped, corrugated narrowing of the bronchial lumen and in-folding of the bronchial mucosa. The bronchial lumen is completely obstructed by tenacious mucus.

LM
Stain: PAS
Magnification: 420:1

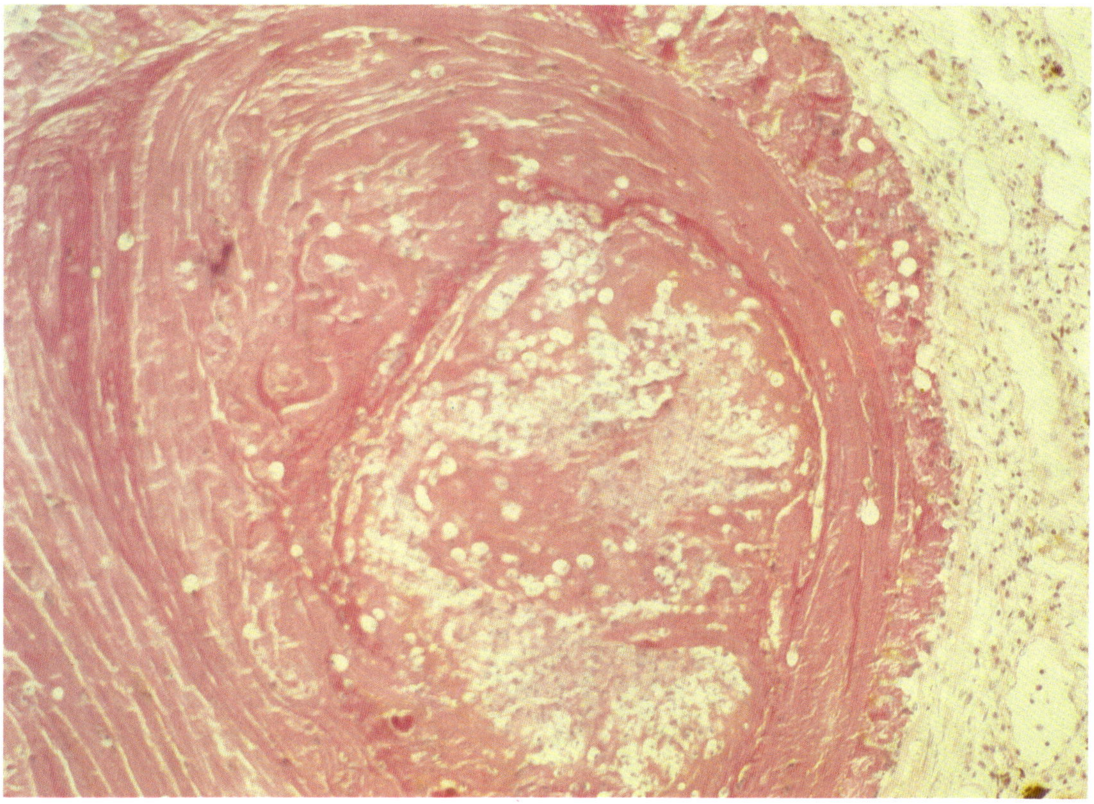

Fig. 80: Bronchial asthma. Complete occlusion of the bronchial lumen with spirally arranged tenacious mucus in a peripheral bronchiole. Only occasional inflammatory cells are present in the secretions.

LM
Stain: PAS
Magnification: 420:1

Fig. 81: Bronchial asthma. Marked hyperplasia of goblet cells in the bronchial epithelium of a mucosal fold. Between the markedly enlarged, secretion-filled goblet cells, only occasional basal cells are seen. Eosinophils are present in the subepithelial connective tissue.

LM
Stain: Hematoxylin-eosin
Magnification: 850:1

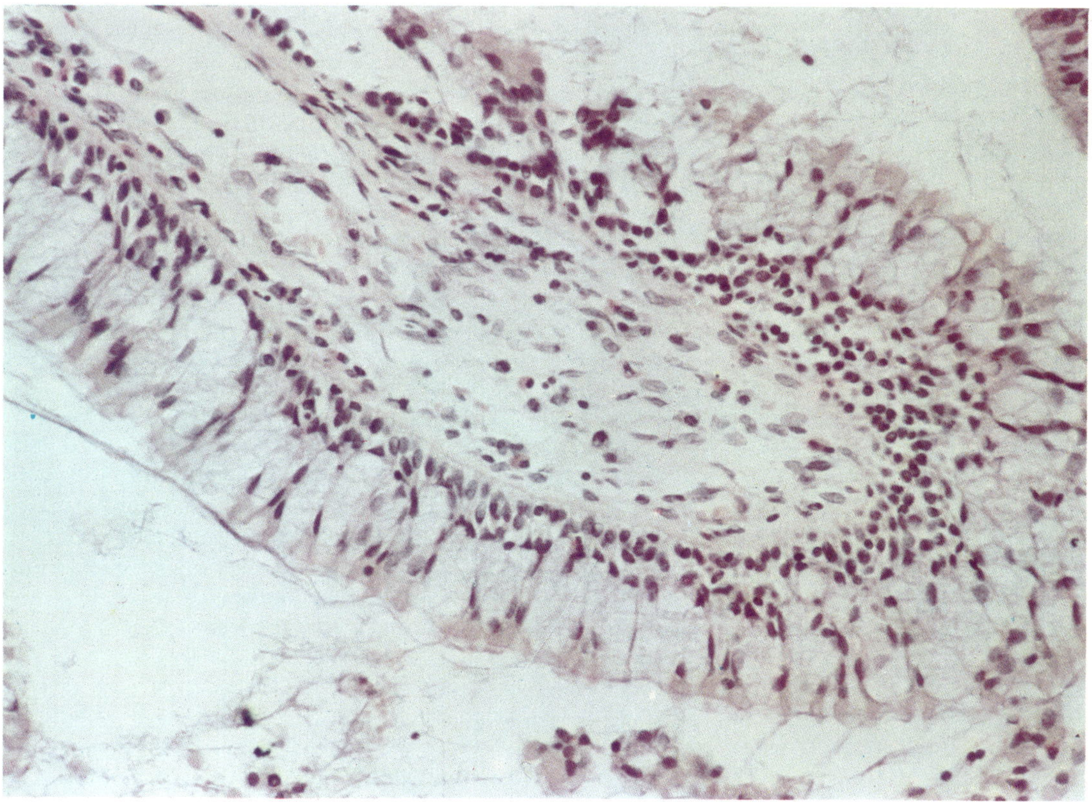

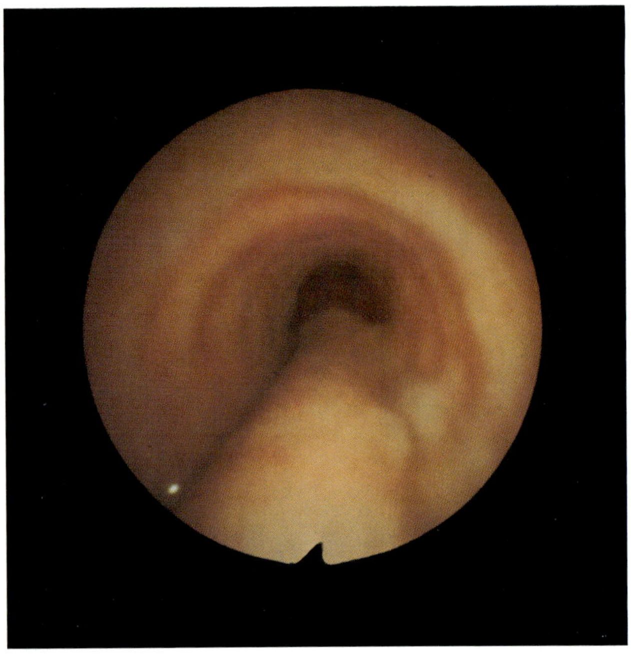

Fig. 82: Cough. Airway instability.
Moderate instability is present resulting in a 40% reduction in airway caliber due to herniation of the pars membranacea into the airway lumen. The mucosa shows focal hypertrophy.

Fig. 83: Cough. Airway instability.
The instability is greater and the lumen is obliterated approximately 60% by pars membranacea herniation. Accumulation of purulent secretions in this situation may lead to life-threatening obstruction.

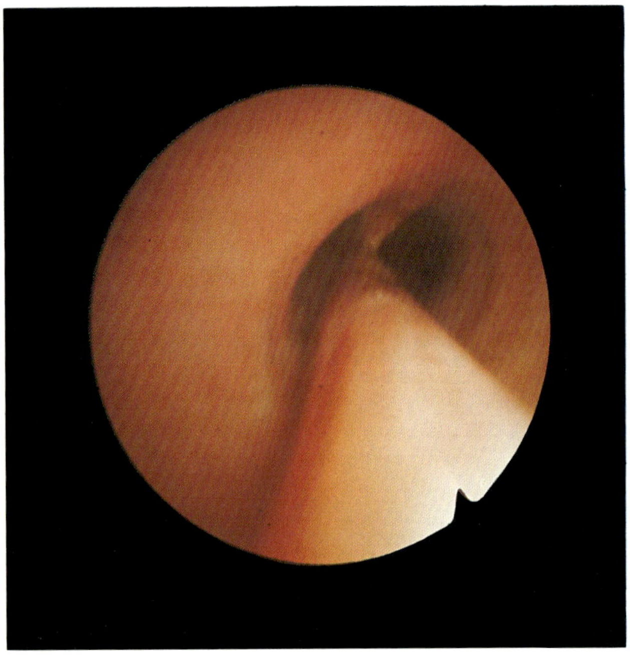

sult of the action of released mediators on bronchial smooth muscle. The bronchus shows corrugated appearance in cross section. Mucosal oedema results from arteriolar constriction, haemostasis and capillary dilatation. Furthermore, there is evidence of increased capillary and epithelial permeability. In addition to hypersecretion, there is increased mucous viscosity and bronchi and bronchioles may become more or less completely obstructed by very viscous mucous casts. When expectorated, these can be seen as small, irregular, sometimes branching, spiral mucous masses, called Curschmann's spirals. These consist of a central basophilically staining core around which mucus is wound in a spiral fashion. The viscous mucus comes from the goblet cells and the peribronchial glands which show hyperplasia and hypertrophy. The goblet cells are almost all in the same stage of secretory hyperactivity and hypersecretion. The goblet cells may even disintegrate resulting in a kind of holocrine secretion. With regression of the acute episode, oedema fluid from the bronchial mucosa may fill the space between the secretions and the bronchial epithelium, facilitating clearance of secretions as a result of cough.

Presumably, it is the release of histamine in the airway wall that results in infiltration of the submucosa by eosinophils. Granulocytes may pass through the surface epithelium to appear in the frequently infected bronchial secretions. These secretions may also contain colourless, Charcot-Leyden crystals derived from disintegrating leukocyte granules. These have a six-sided bipyramidal shape.

The typical clinical appearance of acute asthma is characterized by dyspnea, with more marked expiratory airways obstruction. The thorax appears fixed in inspiration, the shoulders are drawn upwards and the accessory muscles of respiration are mobilized. Patients may be wheezing audibly, while auscultation of the chest may reveal the characteristic wheezing on expiration, and with advancing airways obstruction, on inspiration as well. If airways obstruction is extremely severe, breath sounds may be greatly diminished or absent and adventitious sounds scarce.

Lung function testing shows evidence of more or less severe airways obstruction. The chest X-ray shows evidence of gas trapping and hyperinflation with an increased anteroposterior diameter, widened intercostal spaces, low relatively flat diaphragms and generalized hyperlucency in the peripheral lung fields. All of these changes are reversible with appropriate therapy.

Status asthmaticus is a condition of life-threatening asthma characterized by extremely severe airways obstruction which is not responsive to bronchodilator therapy, but usually requires additional vigourous steroid therapy and occasionally even mechanical ventilatory assistance, while awaiting a beneficial response to steroids.

3.7. Bronchiectasis

Bronchiectasis may be defined as dilatation of large and small bronchi associated with inflammation of the bronchial wall, resulting in irreversible destruction of the wall. By contrast, bronchiectasia consists of dilatation of a relatively normal bronchial wall. Bronchiectasis may be either congential or acquired.

Congenital bronchiectasis may result from partial or complete failure of normal differentiation of the lung. Bronchi terminate blindly in saccular dilatations. Failure of normal development may lead to structural changes in the whole lung or in individual segments. Abnormalities of differentiation of individual bronchi may lead to development of a bronchial cyst.

Acquired bronchiectasis may be divided into saccular and cylindrical types. Saccular bronchiectasis consists of airways terminating in clusters of vesicular cavities originating mainly from medium sized bronchi and rarely extending to the pleura. These changes are seen predominantly in the elderly. This type of bronchiectasis does not tend to progress. The atrophic mucosa frequently shows squamous metaplasia.

In cylindrical bronchiectasis, the bronchi become thick-walled and show progressive dilatation of the lumen from segmental bronchi towards the periphery. The distended small bronchi and bronchioles show destructive hypertrophic or atrophic inflammatory changes. The di-

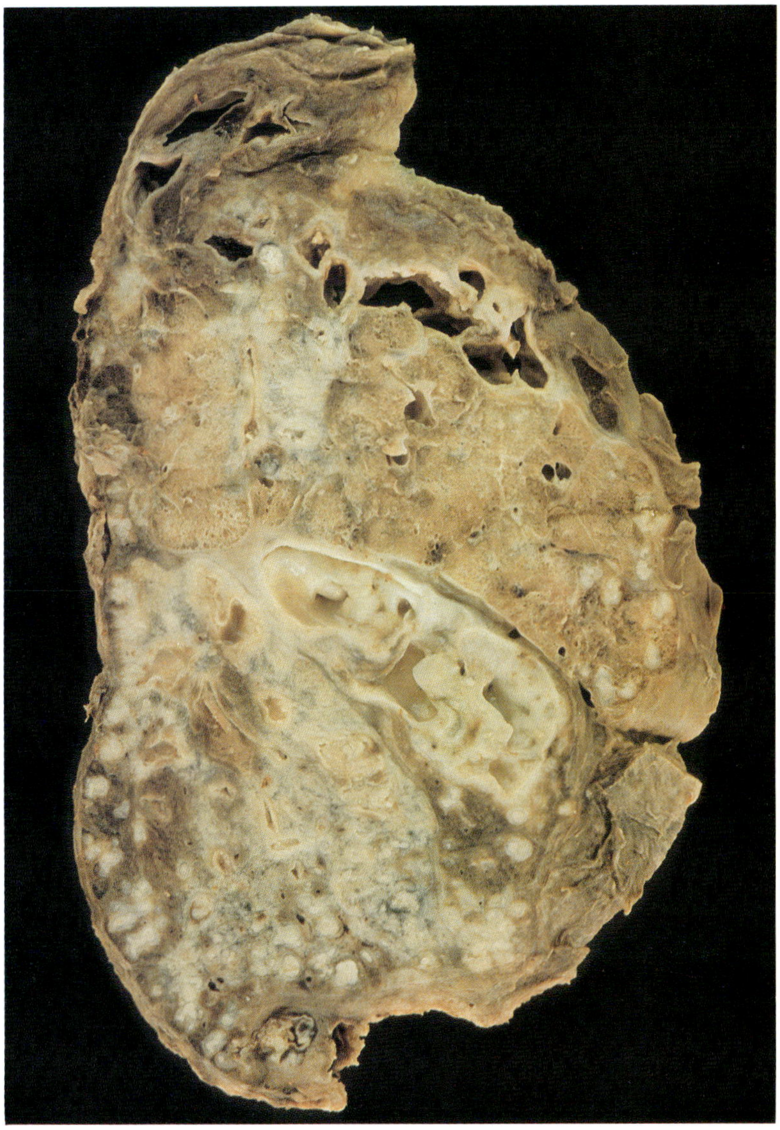

Fig. 84: Bronchiectasis.
Macroscopic appearance of partly cylindrical, partly saccular changes in whole lung section. The markedly dilated bronchi contain accumulations of secretion. Between the widened bronchi, the lung parenchyma shows patchy atelectasis and areas of pneumonitis.

lated airway lumen is filled with tenacious purulent secretions. The smooth muscle and, to some extent, cartilage in the bronchial wall may be destroyed and replaced by scar tissue. The adjacent pulmonary parenchyma shows areas of patchy atelectasis, pneumonitis and fibrosis. Cylindrical bronchiectasis is found mainly in the upper lobes, particularly posteriorly and inferiorly. This form of brochiectasis usually begins in infancy and tends to progress.

Acquired bronchiectasis is mainly the result of retained secretions and superinfection. Failure to eliminate secretions may result from:

- bronchial stenosis in major airways due to inhaled foreign bodies and stenosis secondary to scarring as a result of tuberculosis, fungal infections of the airway, sarcoidosis or endobronchial tumours

- destructive and obliterative bronchitis

- cystic fibrosis

- primary ciliary dyskinesia (Kartagener's syndrome, immotile cilia syndrome).

Fig. 85: Bronchiectasis. Histological appearance.
Variably widened bronchial lumena with marked atrophy of the bronchial mucosa. Peribronchial scarring which extends deeply into the adjacent atelectatic and consolidated lung parenchyma.

LM
Stain: van Gieson
Magnification: 180:1

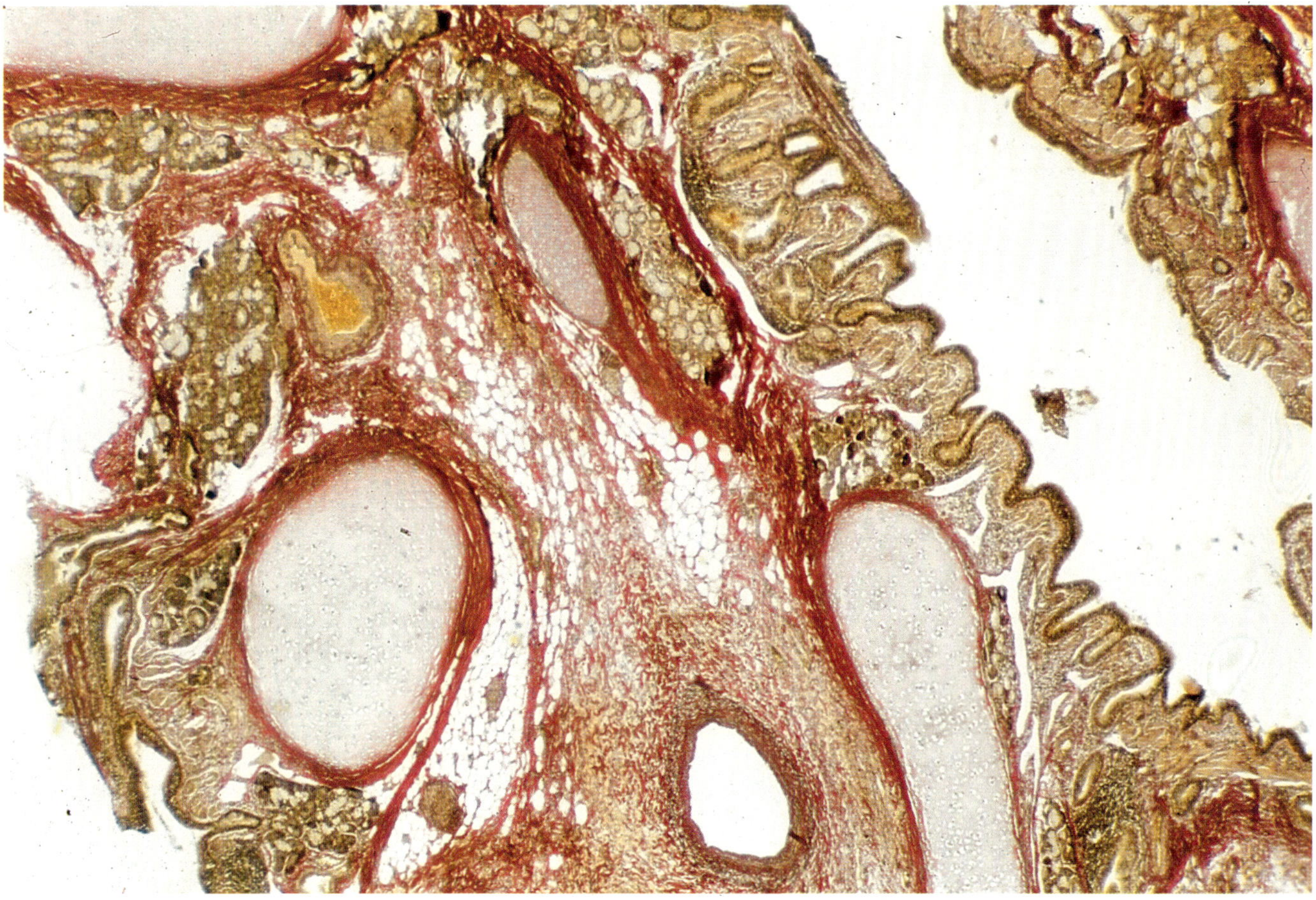

3.8. Primary Ciliary Dyskinesia (Kartagener's Syndrome)

Primary ciliary dyskinesia is a condition characterized clinically by recurring respiratory tract infections, starting in childhood. Typically, the patients present with severe chronic rhinorrhea and sinusitis, serous otitis media and recurring episodes of bronchitis and pneumonia in infancy and childhood, usually resulting in bilateral bronchiectasis. Kartagener's syndrome is a subset of this condition characterized by associated total situs inversus, present in about 50 % of these cases.

The pathophysiological defect consists of grossly abnormal and chaotic ciliary movement or occasionally total absence of ciliary motion (dyskinesia), associated with and likely due to various ultrastructural defects of cilia and sperm evident on electron microscopy. The most common defect so far recognized is absence of dynein arms which are normally attached to subfibre A of the peripheral microtubular doublets of the ciliary ax-

Fig. 86: Bronchial mucosa showing ciliary deficiency.
Marked loss of cilia on the epithelial surface. Tenacious mucus on the surface into which cilia penetrate to varying depths. The cell surface is densely covered with microvilli. The apical portion of the ciliated cell contains many mitochondria reflecting the high metabolic activity.

TEM
Magnification: 12,000:1

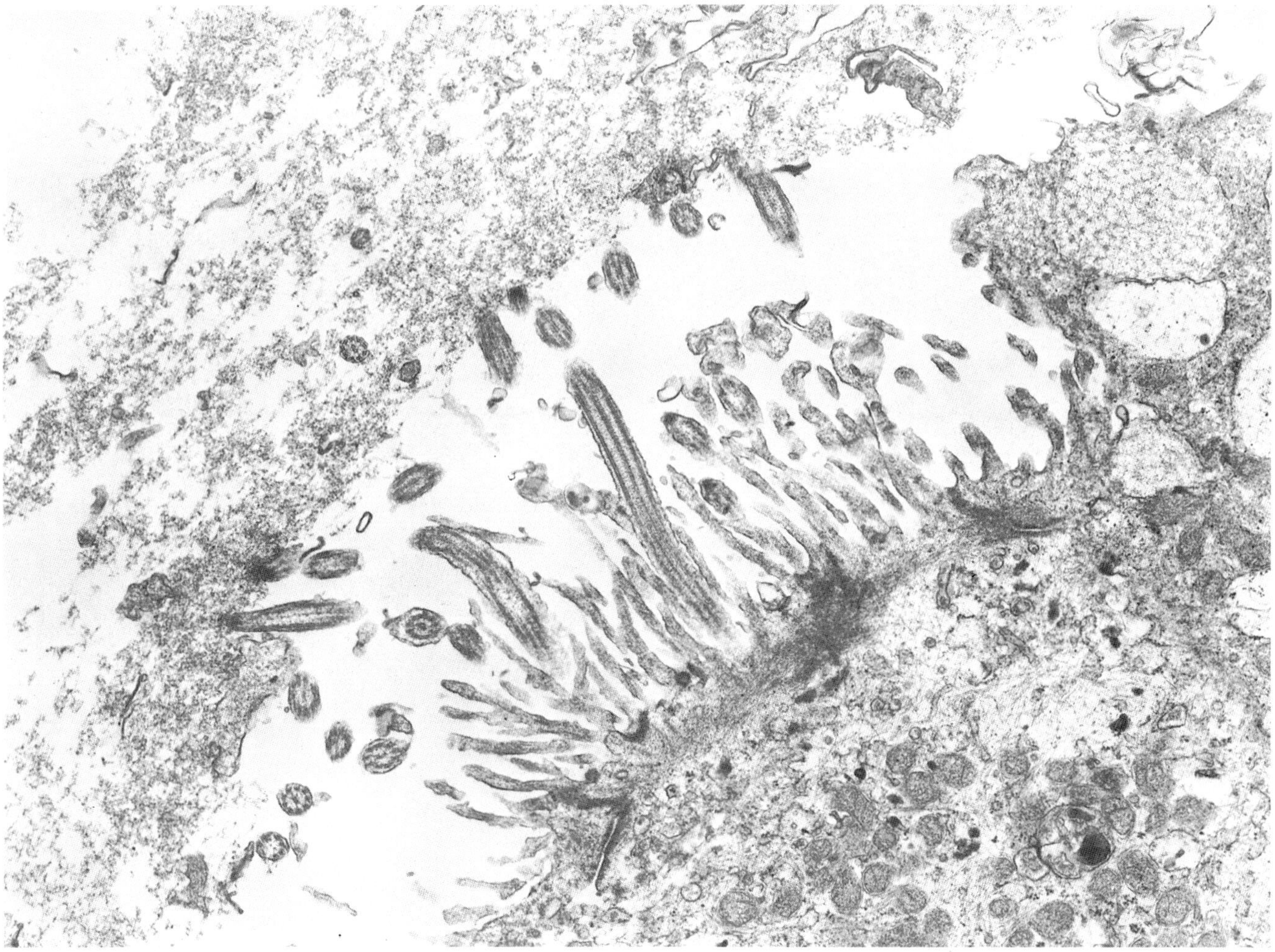

oneme. Less commonly, there may be absent or collapsed radial spokes between the central microtubules and the peripheral doublets. Very rarely, the central tubules may be absent and associated with transposition of peripheral doublets into the central position. Characteristically, the cilia are randomly oriented and this, together with the abnormal wave form invariably seen, results in virtually complete failure of mucociliary transport.

Because sperm have a similar ultrastructure to respiratory tract cilia, sperm motion is also abnormal, resulting in infertility in males with this condition and greatly reduced, although not absent, fertility in females.

While extremely rare (one in 25 - 30,000), primary ciliary dyskinesia should be considered in the differential diagnosis of recurrent respiratory tract infections, chronic bronchitis and bronchiectasis, if the history indicates an onset in infancy or early childhood, and other possible causes, such as asthma or cystic fibrosis have been excluded. It should be possible to establish the diagnosis using nasal or bronchial mucosal biopsy and electron microscopy in experienced hands, the single most important criterion being random orientation of the "feet" of the basal body at the base of the cilia.

Fig. 87a: Primary ciliary dyskinesia (Kartagener's syndrome).
Abnormal ciliary ultrastructure characterized by virtual absence of dynein arms on the peripheral microtubular doublets at three levels (a, b, c) and random orientation of the central microtubules (d). The diagram (e) shows abnormal ultrastructure and (f) illustrates two types of abnormal motion. In this condition cilia beat at half the normal frequency (6 Hz) and mucociliary transport is absent.

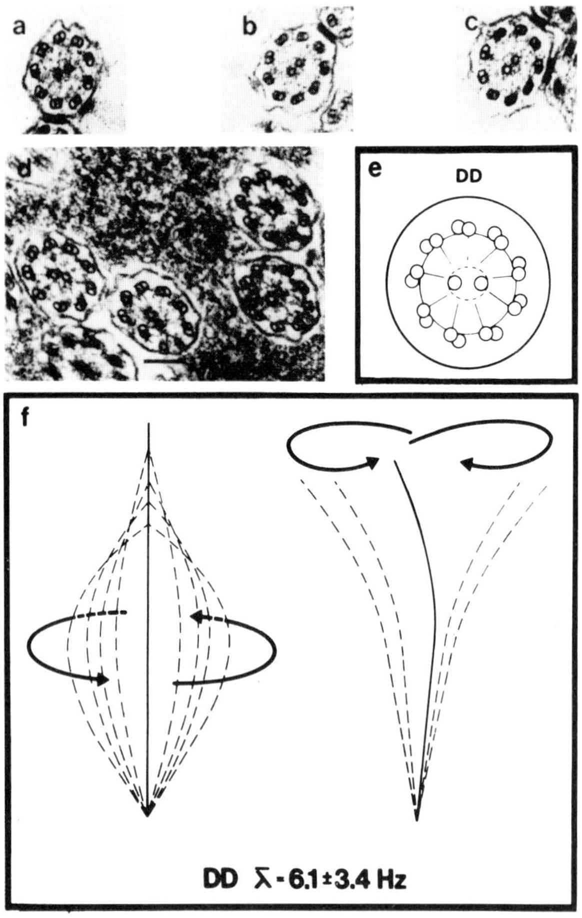

Fig. 87b: Normal ciliary ultrastructure at three levels (a, b, c). Uniform orientation of central microtubules (d). Cilia beat with a normal wave form and frequency (12 Hz).

TEM
Magnification: 50,000:1

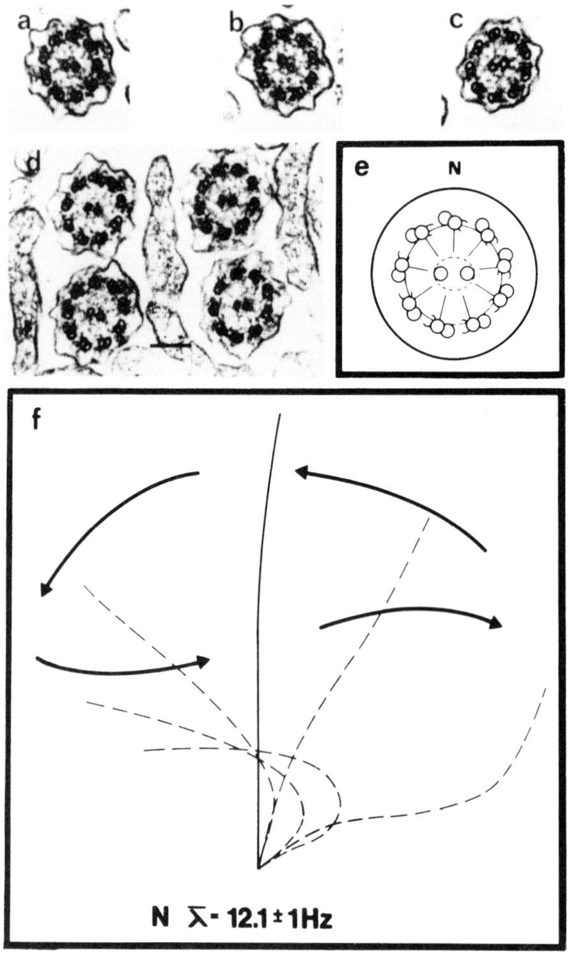

3.9. Tracheomalacia

As a result of prolonged endotracheal intubation or tracheostomy, there may be extensive and marked destruction of the tracheal wall and the adjacent bronchial segments. This results from chronic inflammation secondary to the endotracheal tube and associated infection. Following initial hyperaemia and oedema of the mucosa, mucosal haemorrhage may develop and eventually, with prolonged injury, the mucosa may ulcerate down to the bronchial cartilage. Granulation tissue usually develops in association with the areas of ulcera-

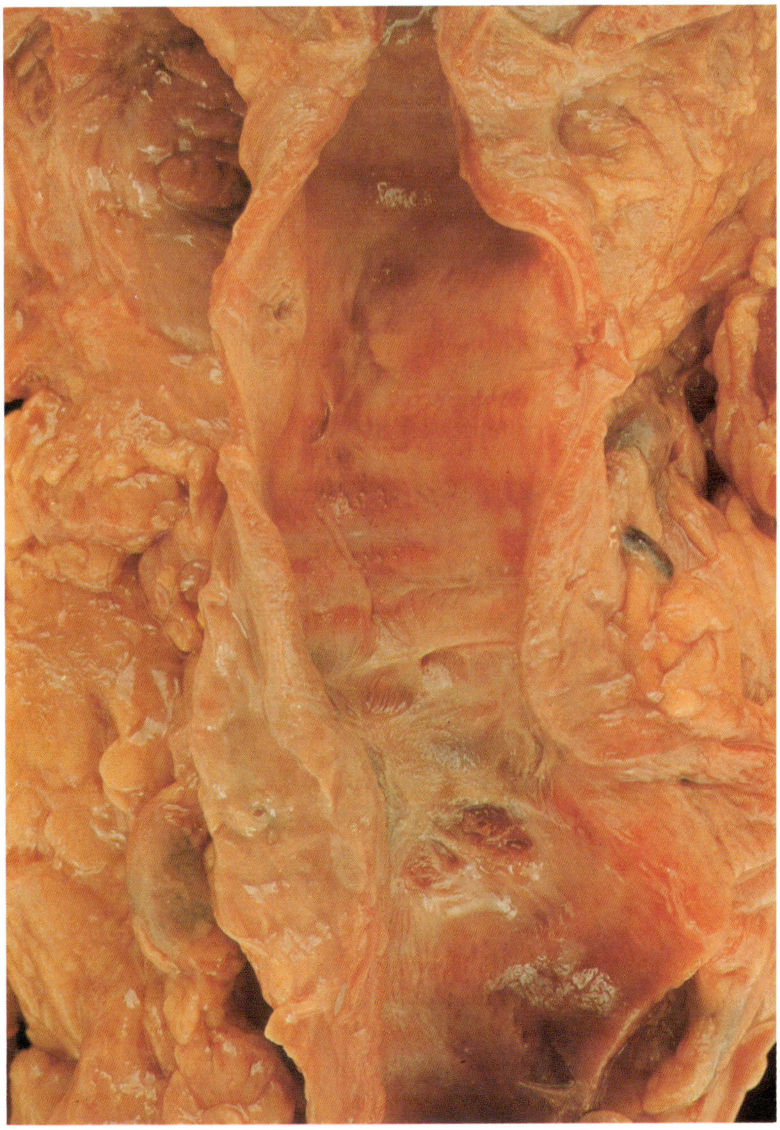

Fig. 88: Severe necrotizing bronchitis with scarring resulting from tracheal wall injury associated with long-term intubation and assisted ventilation. The mucosa shows distortion and there is considerable stenosis of the lumen.

tion. With healing, considerable scar formation may occur, and tracheal or bronchial stenoses may result. The mucosa usually becomes re-epithelialized.

Rarely, idiopathic tracheomalacia may occur due to weakness of the cartilaginous supporting structure particularly in males over 50, which may lead to narrowing of the tracheal lumen in its transvere diameter, while at the same time, there may be an increase in the sagittal diameter. Tracheomalacia may be a congenital condition in the newborn, leading to upper airways obstruction.

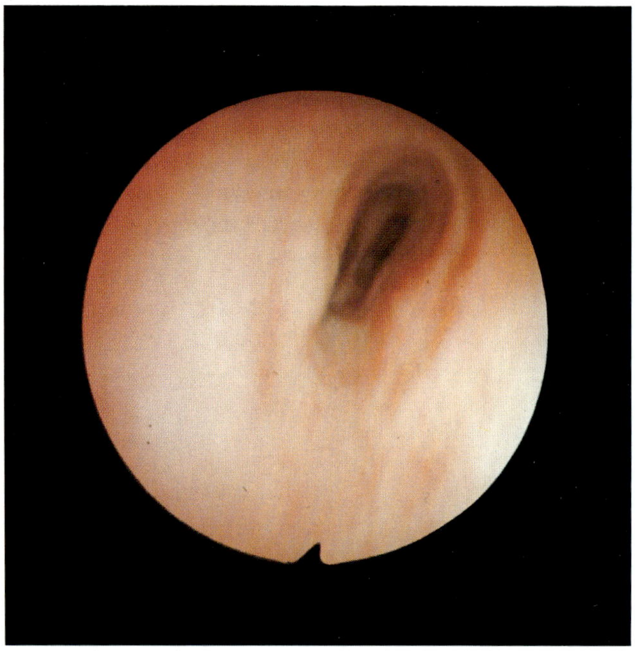

Fig. 89: Tracheomalacia. Sabre scabbard trachea. Softening of the cartilaginous rings leads to a marked reduction of the transverse diameter of the trachea. Vigorous cough causes the free ends of the cartilaginous rings to slam together.

Fig. 90: Localized tracheomalacia. In the centre of the trachea, the right side of one of the rings is pushed inwards. This could indicate early tracheal softening or, alternatively could be the result of external compression by lymph nodes or tumour.

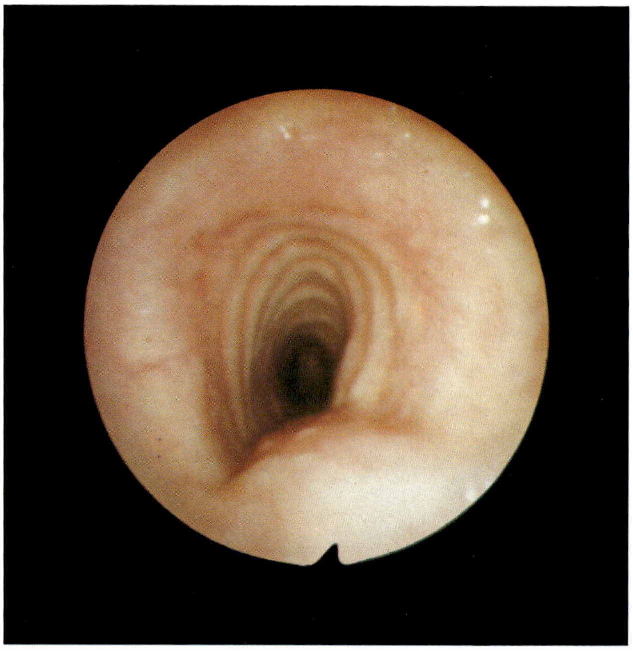

References

Bauer, E.: Zur Biochemie des endobronchialen Fluidsystems. In: Rensch, H., ed.: Mukustransport. Dustri-Verlag Dr. Karl Feistle, München-Deisenhofen, 1980.

Clara, M.: Zur Histologie des Bronchialepithels. Z.mikr.-anat.Forsch. 1937; 41:321-347.

Fletcher, C., Peto, R., Tinker, C., Speizer, F.E.: The Natural History of Chronic Bronchitis and Emphysema. Oxford University Press, Oxford, 1976.

Giese, W.: Atemorgane. In: Staemmler, M., ed.: Lehrbuch der speziellen pathologischen Anatomie. Walther de Gruyter u. Co., Berlin, 1960.

Giese, W.: Atemwege und Lunge. In: Doerr, W., ed.: Organpathologie. Thieme, Stuttgart, 1974.

Götz, H.: Bedeutung der Immunologie im Bereich der Atemwege. Atemwegs-und Lungenkrankheiten 1975; 2:69-80.

Hartung, W.: Pathologische Anatomie der Bronchitis und Bronchiektasie, des Lungenemphysems und der Atelektase. In: Ulmer, W.T., ed.: Handb. der inneren Medizin. Springer, Berlin-Heidelberg-New York, 1979.

Hayek, H. von: Die menschliche Lunge. Springer, Berlin-Heidelberg-New York, 1970.

Morgenroth, K.: Morphological Alterations to the Bronchial Mucosa in High-Dosage Long-Term Exposure to Sulfur Dioxide. Respiration 1980; 39:39-48.

Morgenroth, K., Hoerstebrock, U.: Transmissions- und rasterelektronenmikroskopische Untersuchungen zur Struktur der "Clarazellen" des Bronchialsystems. Arzneimittel-Forsch. Drug Res. 1978; 28:911-917.

Morgenroth, K., Schlake, W.: Unspezifische Begleitreaktion in der Bronchialwand bei der Lungentuberkulose und ihre Behandlung mit NA 872. Wien. med. Wschr. 1975; Suppl. 23.

Morgenroth, K., Nolte, D.: Atlas der Pneumologie. PVG Pharmazeutische Verlagsges., München, 1981.

Morgenroth, K.: Morphologische Aspekte der Sekretion in den kleineren Atemwegen. In: Rensch, H., ed.: Mukustransport. Dustri-Verlag Dr. Karl Feistle, München-Deisenhofen, 1980.

Nilson, B.S., ed.: Scandinavian Symposium on Chronic Obstructive Airways Disease. Scand. J. Respir. Dis. 1979; Suppl. 103.

Reid, L.: Bronchial mucus production in health and disease. In: The Lung. International Academy of Pathology Williams and Wilkins, Baltimore, 1968.

Reid, L.: Evaluation of Model System for Study of Airway Epithelium, Cilia and Mucus. Arch. Intern. Med. 1979; 126:428-434.

Reid, L.: An experimental study of hypersecretion of mucus in bronchial tree. Brit. J. Exp. Path. 1963; 44:437-445.

Rossman, C.M., Forrest, J.B., Lee, R.M.K.W., Newhouse, A.F., Newhouse, M.T.: The Dyskinetic Cilia Syndrome. Abnormal Ciliary Motility in Association with Abnormal Ciliary Ultrastructure. Chest 1981; 805:860-864.

Rossman, C.M., Lee, R.M.K.W., Forrest, J.B., Newhouse, M.T.: Nasal Cilia in Normal Man, Primary Ciliary Dyskinesia and Other Respiratory Diseases: Analysis of Motility and Ultrastructure. Europ.J. Respir. Dis.(in press).

Spencer, H.: Pathology of the Lung. Pergamon Press, Oxford, New York, Toronto, Sydney, Paris, Frankfurt, 1977.

PVG Pharmazeutische Verlagsgesellschaft publishes a series of atlases of pathology which include three-dimensional diagrams to illustrate gross and microscopic anatomy.

Further titles:

Morgenroth, Newhouse, Nolte
Atlas of Pulmonary Pathology

Holzner, Mathes, Metzenbauer, Baxley
Atlas of Heart Disease

Mathes, Gehring
Cardiac Rhythm Disorders

Ottenjann, Altaras, Elster, Hermanek
Atlas of Intestinal Disease

Morgenroth, Hildmann, Pucher
Rhino-Sinusitis

Mathies, Richter
Arthritis

Mondorf
Atlas of Renal Disease

Mathies, Richter
Arthrosis

Morgenroth, Kronberger
Pneumoconioses

Morgenroth
Venous thrombosis

Reichart, Weinhold
Surgical Treatment of Heart Disease

Morgenroth
Bronchial Asthma

Karrer, Hermanek
Tumours I

Koos
Cerebral Hemorrhage

Koos
Cerebral Emergency

Morgenroth, Herzog, Opferkuch
Pneumonia

Bandmann
Atlas of Dermatology

English Edition:
Butterworth Scientific Ltd.
Borough Green, Sevenoaks, Kent TN15 8PH
Telephone: (0732) 884567
Telex: 95678
England